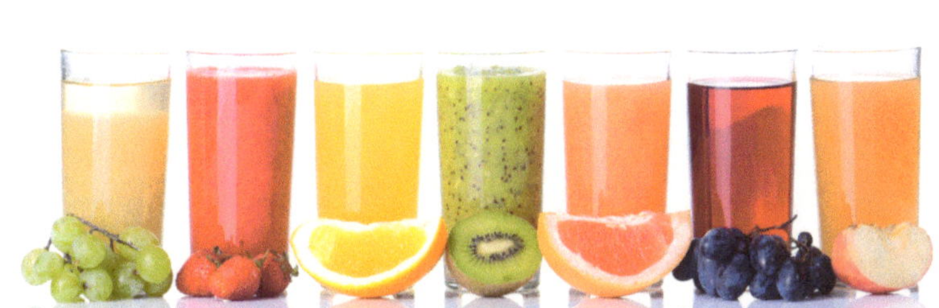

Content

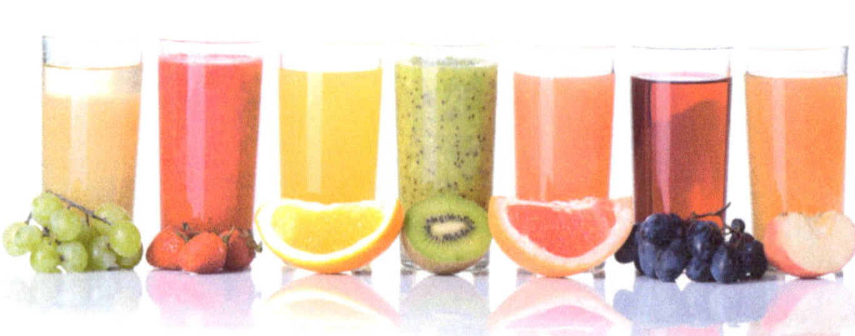

1-6. Stress-Relieving Juices:
Natural relaxation in every sip

In a hectic world, it's more important than ever to find ways to calm your body and mind. Stress-relieving juices offer a soothing way to tackle everyday life with more calm.

These special juices are made from natural ingredients such as calming lavender, relaxing chamomile tea, vitamin-rich spinach and refreshing lemon balm extract.

Rich in antioxidants, vitamins and minerals, they support stress management while promoting general well-being.

Enjoy this gentle but effective relaxation aid that helps you find inner peace - simply by taking a delicious sip.

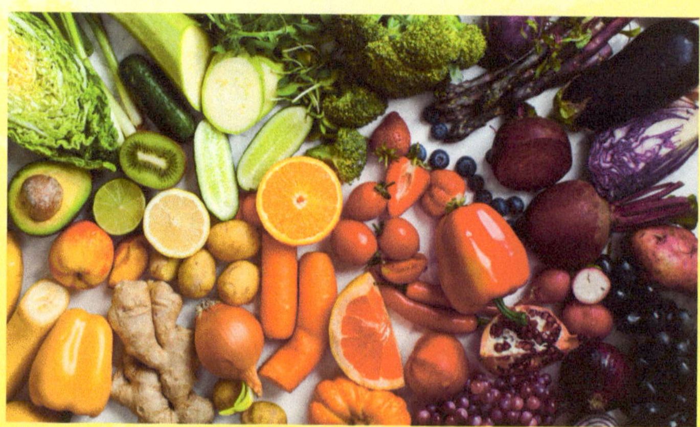

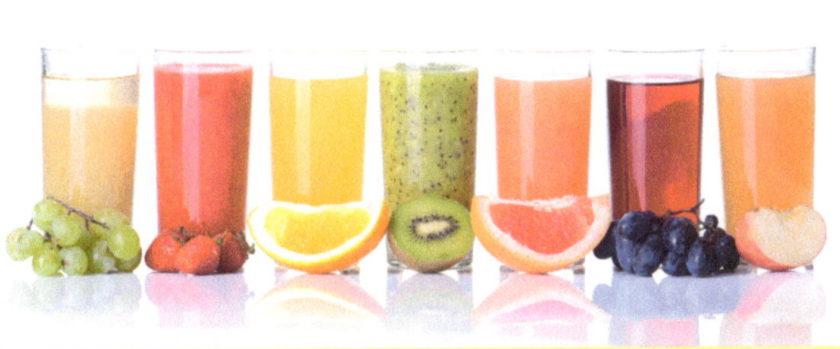

1. Kale and cucumber juice (1000 ml)

Ingredients:
- 150 g kale (approx. 3-4 large leaves)
- 1 large cucumber (approx. 300 g)
- 2 stalks celery (approx. 150 g), parsley to taste
- 2 medium-sized apples (approx. 300 g)
- 1 lemon (juiced, approx. 3-4 tbsp lemon juice)
- 200 ml water* (or as needed to achieve the desired consistency)

Preparation:
1. Prepare the kale: Remove the tough stems and roughly chop the leaves.
2. Prepare the cucumber and celery: Peel the cucumber (optional) and cut it into pieces.
Also cut the celery stalks into smaller pieces.
3. Prepare the apples: Core the apples and cut them into quarters.
4. Blend: Place the kale, cucumber, celery, parsley and apples in a high-powered blender or juicer. Add the lemon juice and water.
5. Blend and strain (optional): Blend until smooth. If you prefer a finer texture, you can strain the juice through a sieve.
6. Serve: Pour the juice into a glass and enjoy fresh.
This recipe makes about 1000 ml of soothing kale and cucumber juice, which is rich in magnesium and relaxes the body.

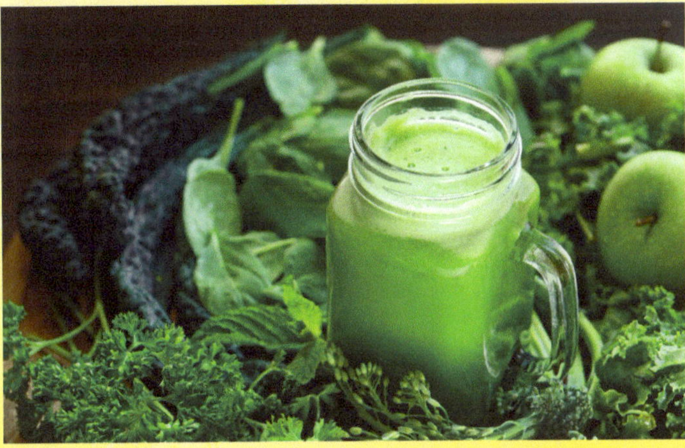

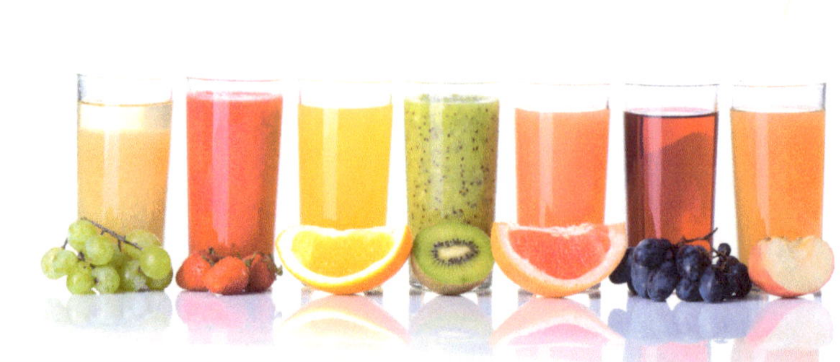

2. Lavender-lemon juice (1000 ml)

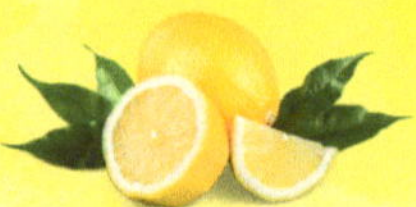

Ingredients:
- 5 lemons (approx. 250 ml lemon juice)
- 4 medium-sized apples (approx. 600 g)
- 2 tsp dried lavender flowers (or 1 tbsp fresh lavender flowers)
- 2-3 tbsp honey (depending on desired sweetness)
-200 ml water (for diluting and for the lavender infusion)
- Ice cubes (optional to cool the juice)

Preparation:

1. Lavender infusion: Boil 200 ml of water and pour it over the lavender flowers. Let the mixture steep for 5-10 minutes, then strain and remove the lavender flowers. Let the lavender infusion cool.
2. Juice the lemons: Squeeze the lemons to get about 250 ml of lemon juice.
3. Juice the apples: Core the apples and juice them to obtain about 500 ml of apple juice.
4. Mix: In a large jug, mix the lemon juice, apple juice and the cooled lavender infusion. Add the honey and stir until completely dissolved.
5. Dilute: Add a little more water if necessary to achieve the desired consistency and adjust the taste.
6. Serve: Pour the juice into a glass, add ice cubes if desired and enjoy fresh.

This recipe yields about 1000 ml of lavender-lemon juice, ideal for relaxing due to the calming effects of lavender.

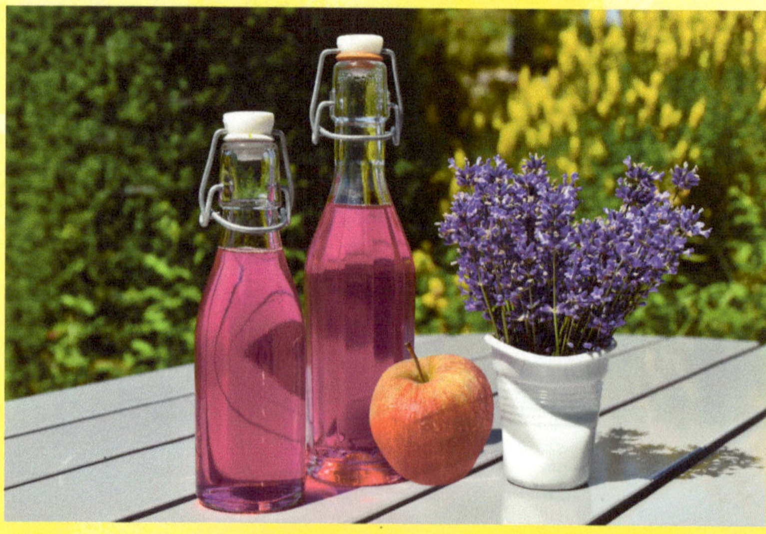

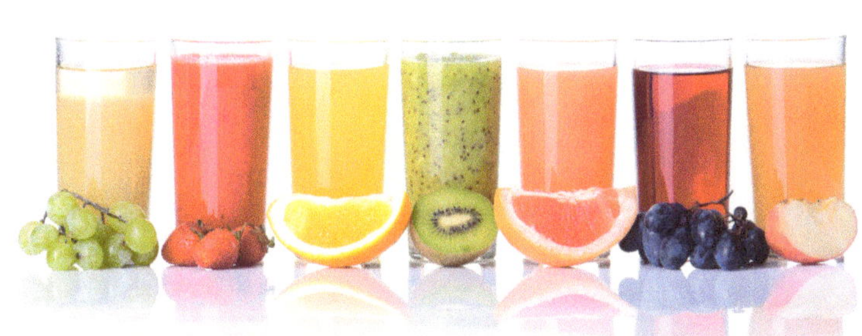

3. Chamomile cucumber juice (1000 ml)

Ingredients:
- 500 ml chamomile tea (strongly brewed and cooled)
- 1 medium cucumber (approx. 200 g), peeled and cut into pieces
- 2 stalks celery (approx. 150 g), washed and cut into pieces
- 10 fresh mint leaves
- 150 ml water (depending on desired consistency)
- Optional: 1-2 tsp honey or another sweetener of choice

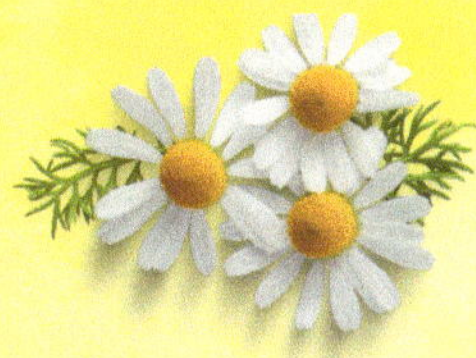

Preparation:
1. Prepare the chamomile tea, let it cool.
2. Peel the cucumber and cut it into pieces.
3. Cut the celery into pieces.
4. Put the cucumber pieces, celery, mint leaves and cooled chamomile tea in a blender.
5. Blend everything until it has a smooth consistency. Add water if necessary to achieve the desired consistency.
6. Optionally, you can season the juice with honey or another sweetener.
7. Strain the juice through a fine sieve or a cloth to obtain a clear liquid.
8. Serve cold.

This recipe makes about 1000 ml of chamomile cucumber juice, which supports stress reduction through vitamin C and antioxidants.

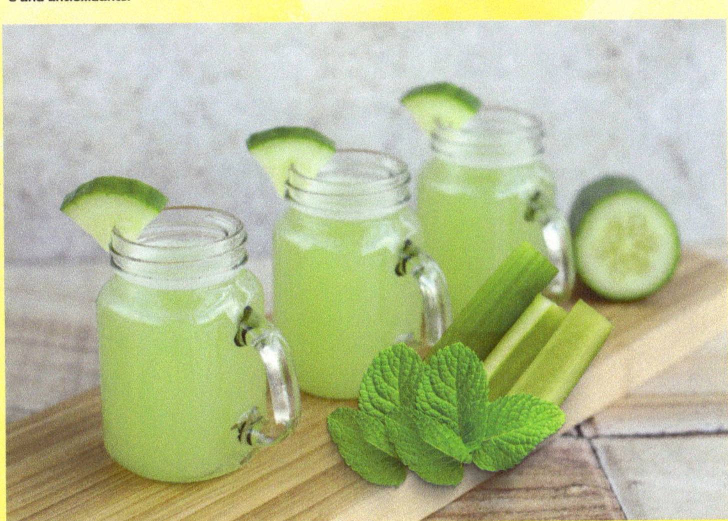

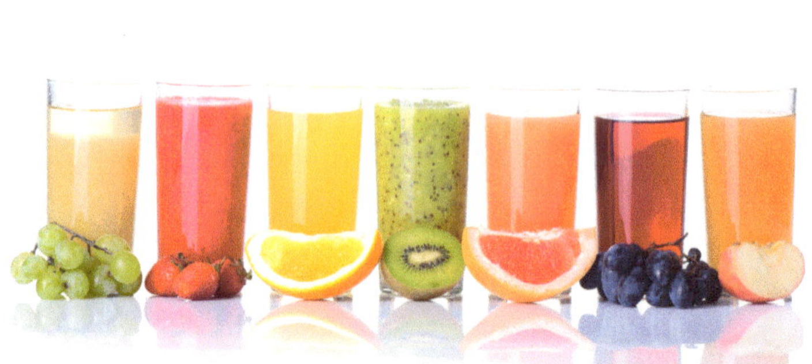

4. Spinach-Pineapple-Juice

Ingredients:
- 200 g fresh spinach, washed
- 300 g fresh pineapple, peeled and cut into pieces
- Juice of 1 lemon (approx. 50 ml)
- 1 small piece of ginger (approx. 10 g), peeled
- 200 ml water (depending on the desired consistency)
- Optional: 1-2 teaspoons honey or other sweetener of your choice

Preparation:
1. Wash the spinach thoroughly.
2. Peel the pineapple and cut it into pieces.
3. Peel the ginger.
4. Put the spinach, pineapple pieces, lemon juice and ginger in a blender.
5. Blend until smooth, adding water if necessary to reach desired consistency.
6. Optionally, you can season the juice with honey or another sweetener.
7. Strain the juice through a fine sieve or cloth to obtain a clear liquid.
8. Serve cold.

This recipe makes about 1000 ml of spinach pineapple juice, which is an ideal source of nutrients and good for stress relief.

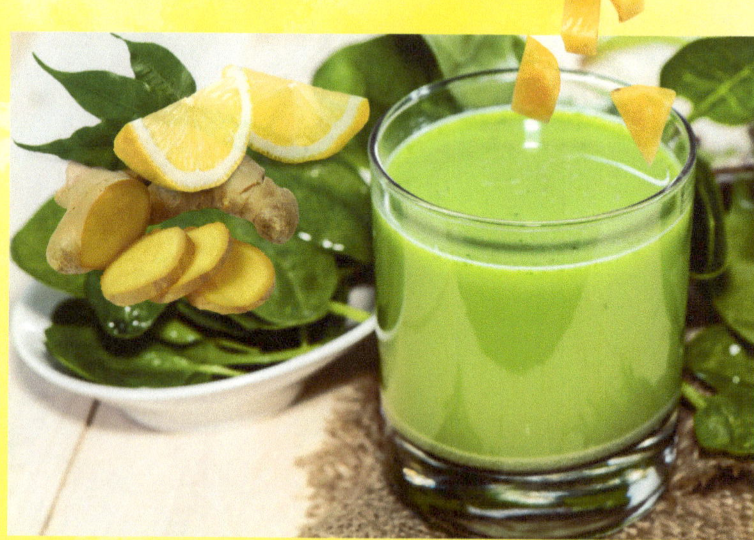

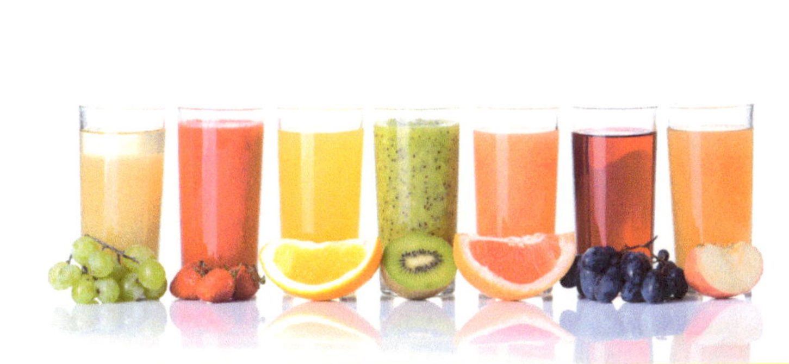

5. Celery green tea juice

Ingredients:
- 2 sticks of celery (approx. 150 g), washed and cut into pieces
- 2 medium-sized apples (approx. 300 g), cored and cut into pieces
- 500 ml green tea (strongly brewed and cooled)
- Juice of 2 limes (approx. 50 ml)
- 100 ml water (depending on the desired consistency)
- Optional: 1-2 teaspoons honey or other sweetener of your choice

Preparation:
1. Prepare the green tea and let it cool.
2. Cut the celery into pieces.
3. Core the apples and cut them into pieces.
4. Place the celery pieces, apple pieces, lime juice and cooled green tea in a blender.
5. Blend until smooth, adding water if necessary to reach desired consistency.
6. Optionally, you can season the juice with honey or another sweetener.
7. Strain the juice through a fine sieve or cloth to obtain a clear liquid.
8. Serve cold.

This recipe makes about 1000 ml of celery green tea juice, which combines the calming properties of green tea with the fresh flavors of celery, apple and lime.

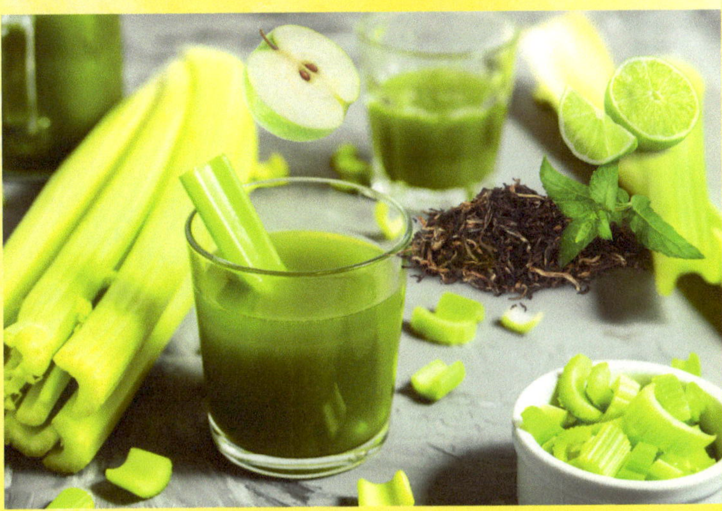

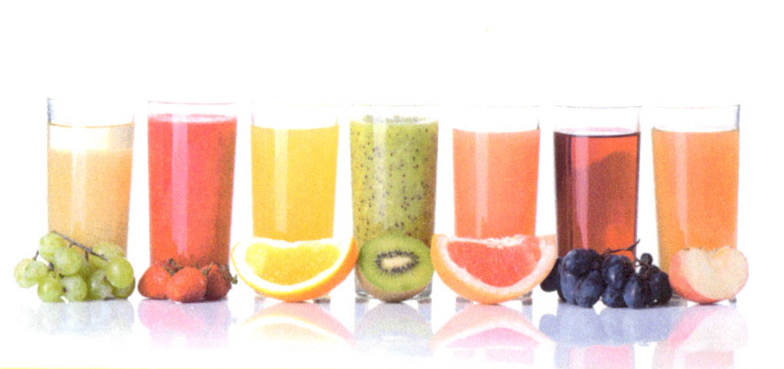

6. Basil-orange juice (1000 ml)

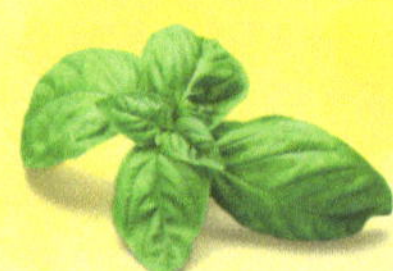

Ingredients:
- 4 large oranges (approx. 600 ml freshly squeezed orange juice)
- 1 large carrot (approx. 100 g), peeled and cut into pieces
- Juice of 2 limes (approx. 50 ml)
- 10 fresh basil leaves
- 200 ml water (depending on the desired consistency)
- Optional: 1-2 teaspoons honey or other sweetener of your choice

Preparation:
1. Squeeze the oranges to obtain about 600 ml of fresh orange juice.
2. Peel the carrot and cut it into pieces.
3. Place the carrot pieces, lime juice, basil leaves and orange juice in a blender.
4. Blend until smooth. Add water if necessary to reach desired consistency.
5. Optionally, you can season the juice with honey or another sweetener.
6. Strain the juice through a fine sieve or cloth to obtain a clear liquid.
7. Serve cold.

This recipe yields about 1000 ml of basil-orange juice, which combines the calming effects of basil and the fresh taste of fruit, ideal for relaxing moments.

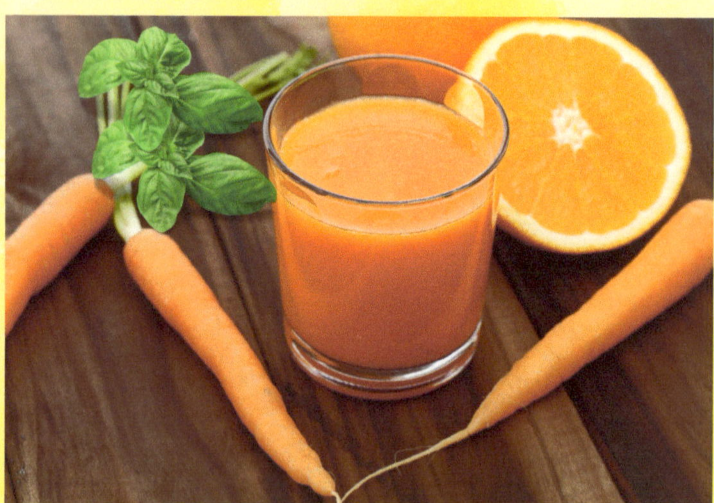

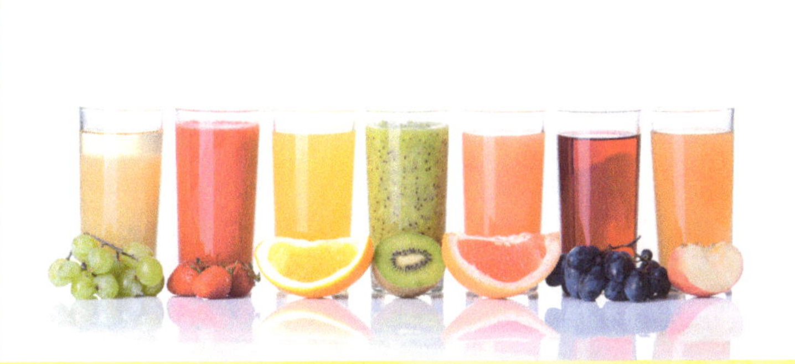

7.-12. Juices for skin improvement:
Radiant skin from within

Radiant, healthy skin starts from within - and our skin improvement juices are the perfect companion on the way to a fresh complexion. These juices are rich in skin-friendly vitamins, minerals and antioxidants that nourish and protect the skin.

With ingredients such as cell-protecting pomegranate, moisturizing cucumber, skin-clarifying aloe vera and antioxidant vitamin C from oranges, they support skin regeneration and promote a natural glow.

Regular consumption of these juices helps to improve the complexion, moisturize and reduce the appearance of blemishes – for healthy, radiant skin that glows from within.

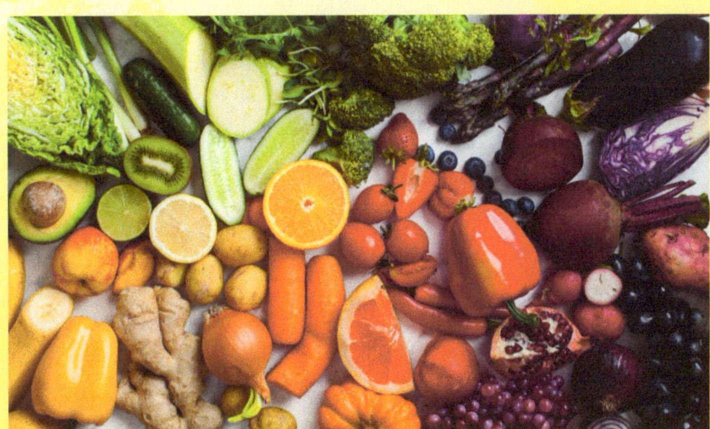

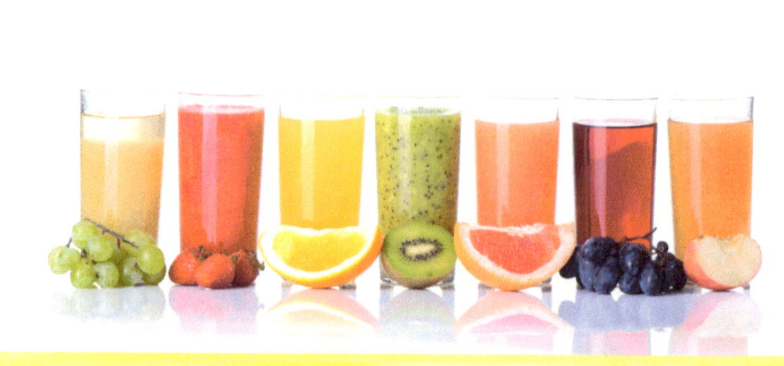

7. Carrot-apple-ginger juice (1000 ml)

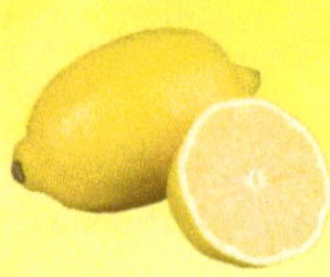

Ingrediance:
- 4 large carrots (approx. 300 g), peeled and cut into pieces
- 2 medium-sized apples (approx. 300 g), cored and cut into pieces
- 1 small piece of ginger (approx. 10 g), peeled
- Juice of 2 lemons (approx. 50 ml)
- 350 ml water (depending on the desired consistency)
- Optional: 1-2 teaspoons honey or other sweetener of your choice

Preparation:
1. Peel the carrots and cut them into pieces.
2. Core the apples and cut them into pieces.
3. Peel the piece of ginger.
4. Put the carrot pieces, apple pieces, lemon juice and ginger in a blender.
5. Blend until smooth, adding water if necessary to reach desired consistency.
6. Optionally, you can season the juice with honey or another sweetener.
7. Strain the juice through a fine sieve or cloth to obtain a clear liquid.
8. Serve cold.

This recipe makes about 1000 ml of carrot-apple-ginger juice, which provides healthy skin with beta-carotene and vitamin C.

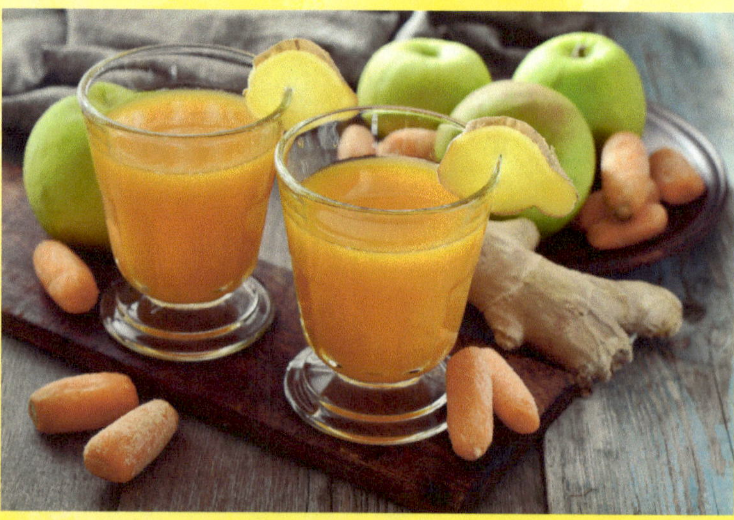

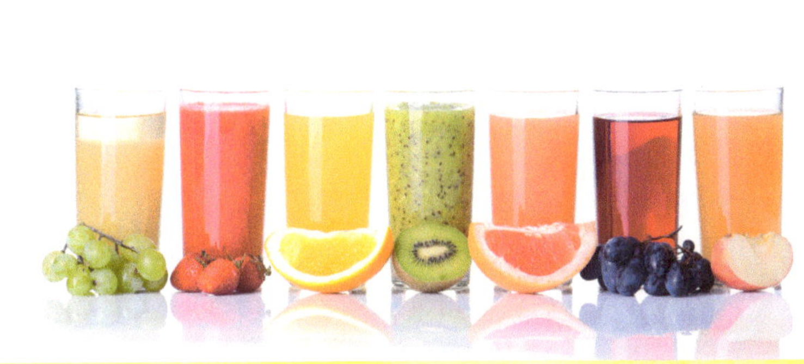

8. Cucumber-mint-lime juice (1000 ml)

Ingredients:
- 1 large cucumber (approx. 300 g), peeled and cut into pieces
- 1 green apple (approx. 150 g), cored and cut into pieces
- Juice of 3 limes (approx. 75 ml)
- 15 fresh mint leaves
- 400 ml water (depending on the desired consistency)
- Optional: 1-2 teaspoons honey or other sweetener of your choice

Preparation:
1. Peel the cucumber and cut it into pieces.
2. Core the green apple and cut it into pieces.
3. Place the cucumber pieces, apple pieces, lime juice and mint leaves in a blender.
4. Blend until smooth. Add water if necessary to reach desired consistency.
5. Optionally, you can season the juice with honey or another sweetener.
6. Strain the juice through a fine sieve or cloth to obtain a clear liquid.
7. Serve cold.

This recipe makes about 1000 ml of cucumber-mint-lime juice, which is ideal for the skin as it is hydrating and refreshing. Perfect on hot days or as a healthy skin booster!

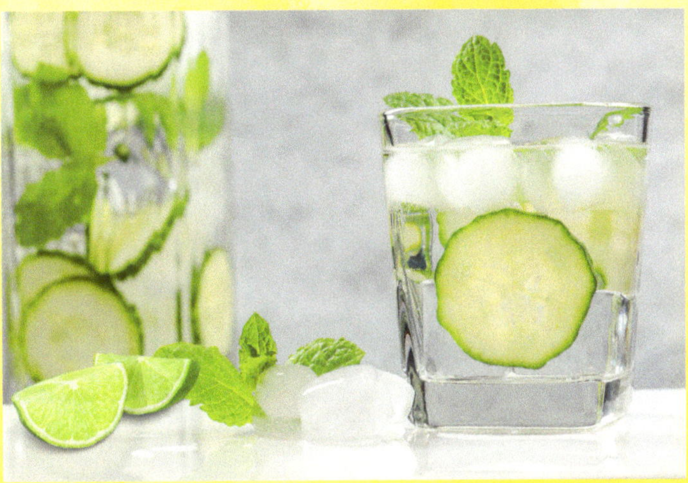

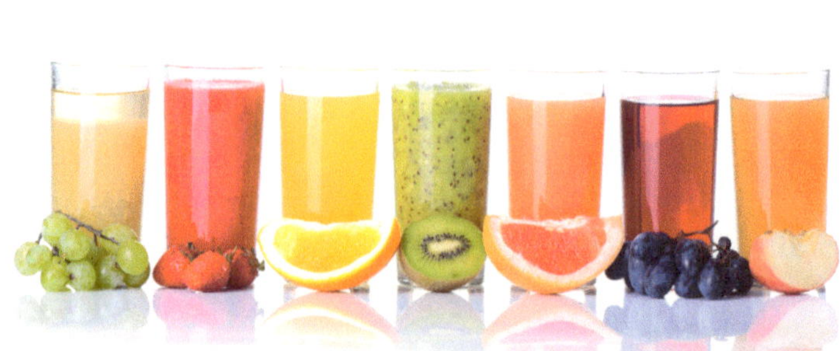

9. Beetroot-orange juice (1000 ml)

Ingredients:
- 1 medium-sized beetroot (approx. 150 g), peeled and cut into pieces
- 3 large oranges (approx. 450 ml freshly squeezed orange juice)
- 2 large carrots (approx. 150 g), peeled and cut into pieces
- 1 small piece of ginger (approx. 10 g), peeled
- 250 ml water (depending on the desired consistency)
- Optional: 1-2 teaspoons honey or other sweetener of your choice

Preparation:
1. Peel the beetroot and cut it into pieces.
2. Squeeze the oranges to obtain about 450 ml of fresh orange juice.
3. Peel the carrots and cut them into pieces.
4. Peel the piece of ginger.
5. Put the beetroot, carrot pieces, orange juice and ginger in a blender.
6. Blend until smooth. Add water if necessary to reach desired consistency.
7. Optionally, you can season the juice with honey or another sweetener.
8. Strain the juice through a fine sieve or cloth to obtain a clear liquid.
9. Serve cold.

This recipe makes about 1000 ml of beetroot and orange juice, which promotes skin elasticity and gives the skin a natural glow thanks to the rich nutrients. Perfect for radiant skin!

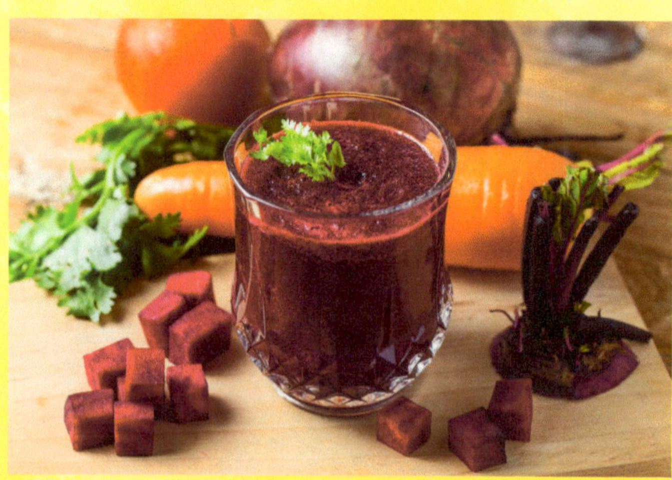

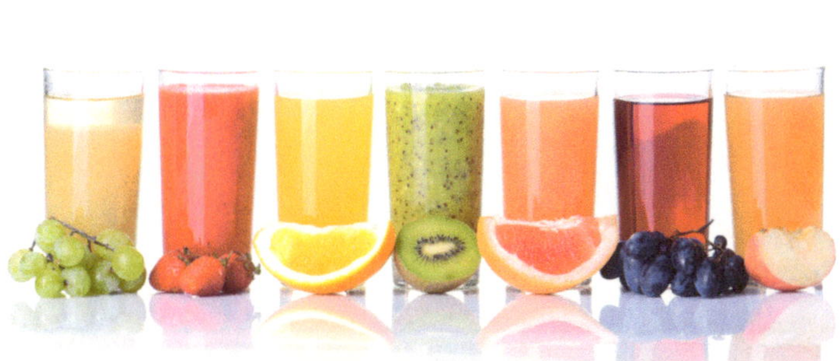

10. Aloe Vera Kiwi Juice (1000 ml)

Ingredients:
- 2-3 leaves of aloe vera (approx. 100 ml aloe vera gel)
- 3 ripe kiwis (approx. 150 g), peeled and cut into pieces
- 1 large cucumber (approx. 200 g), peeled and cut into pieces
- Juice of 3 limes (approx. 75 ml)
- 475 ml water (depending on desired consistency)
- Optional: 1-2 teaspoons honey or other sweetener of your choice

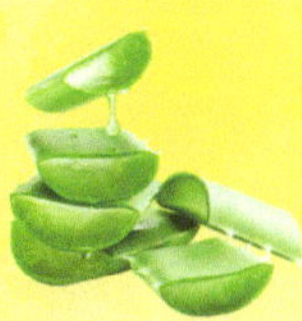

Preparation:
1. Cut the aloe vera leaves and scrape out the gel until you have about 100 ml of gel.
2. Peel the kiwis and cut them into pieces.
3. Peel the cucumber and cut it into pieces.
4. Put the aloe vera gel, kiwi pieces, cucumber pieces and lime juice in a blender.
5. Blend until smooth, adding water if necessary to reach desired consistency.
6. Optionally, you can season the juice with honey or another sweetener.
7. Strain the juice through a fine sieve or cloth to obtain a clear liquid.
8. Serve cold.

This recipe makes about 1000 ml of aloe vera kiwi juice, which combines the healing and soothing properties of aloe vera with the fruity freshness for healthy and radiant skin!

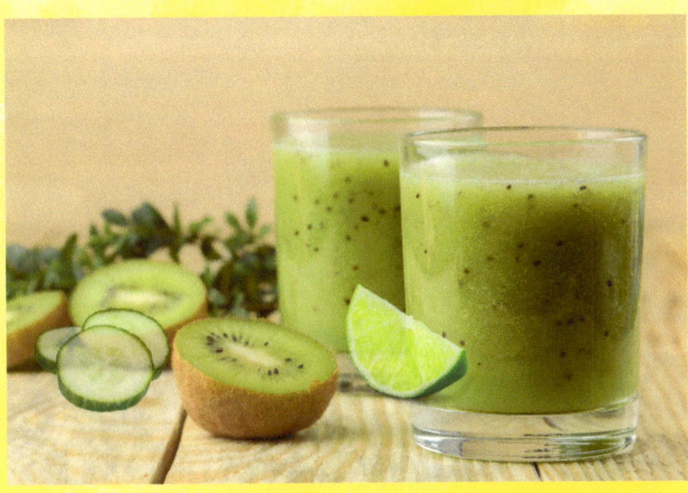

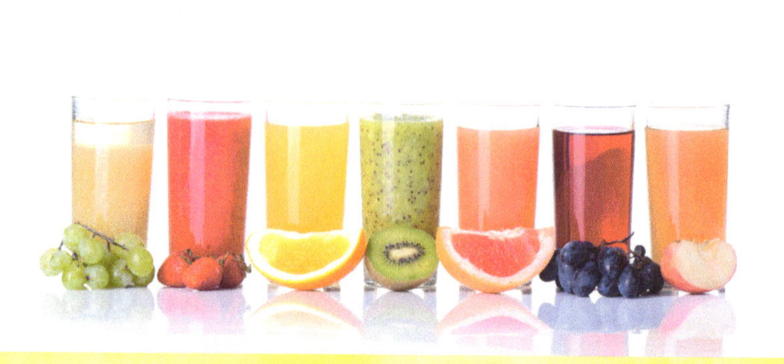

11. Papaya-Mango-Turmeric Juice (1000 ml)

Ingredients:
- 1 small papaya (approx. 300 g), peeled, pitted and cut into pieces
- 1 ripe mango (approx. 300 g), peeled and cut into pieces
- 1 teaspoon fresh turmeric (approx. 5 g), peeled and finely grated (alternatively: ½ teaspoon turmeric powder)
- Juice of 2 limes (approx. 50 ml)
- 350 ml water (depending on the desired consistency)
- Optional: 1-2 teaspoons honey or other sweetener of your choice

Preparation:
1. Peel the papaya and mango, remove the seeds and cut them into pieces.
2. Peel the fresh turmeric and grate it finely (or use turmeric powder).
3. Place the papaya pieces, mango pieces, grated turmeric and lime juice in a blender.
4. Blend until smooth. Add water if necessary to reach desired consistency.
5. Optionally, you can season the juice with honey or another sweetener.
6. Strain the juice through a fine sieve or cloth to obtain a clear liquid.
7. Serve cold.

This recipe makes about 1000 ml of papaya-mango-turmeric juice, which is rich in antioxidants and vitamins that ensure a radiant complexion.

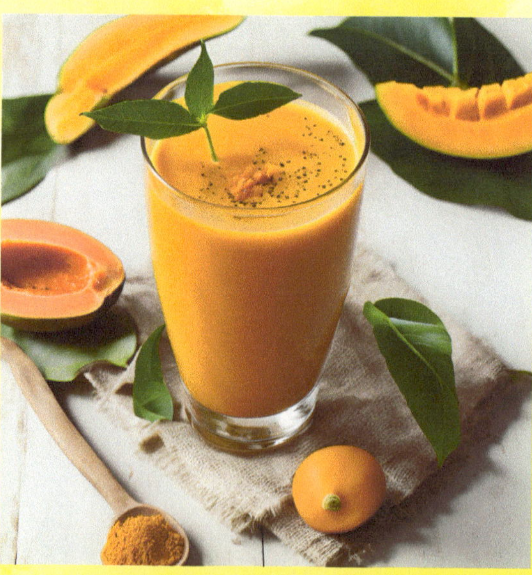

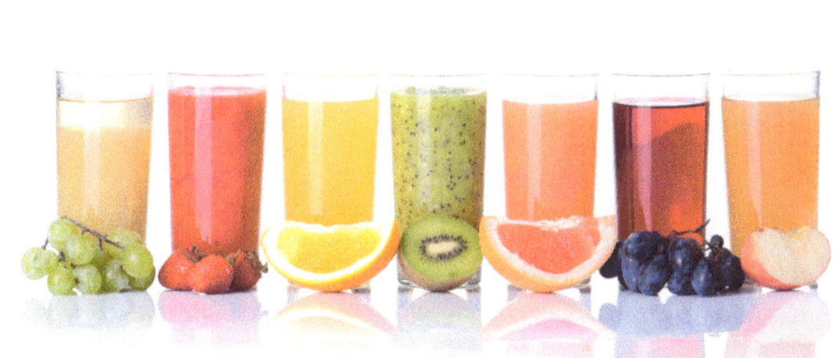

12. Pomegranate-Apple Juice (1000 ml)

Ingredients:
- 2 large pomegranates (about 2 cups of pomegranate seeds)
- 4 medium-sized apples (preferably sweeter varieties such as Gala or Fuji)
- 1 whole lemon (juice)
- 10-12 fresh mint leaves
- Optional: 2-3 tablespoons honey** (to taste)

Preparation:
1. Deseed the pomegranate: Remove the pomegranate seeds from the fruit. You should have about 2 cups of pomegranate seeds.
2. Prepare the apples: Wash the apples, core them and cut them into pieces.
3. Squeeze the lemon: Squeeze the juice from the whole lemon.
4. Blend everything: Put the pomegranate seeds, apple pieces, lemon juice and mint leaves in a powerful blender. Blend everything well until the mixture has a uniform consistency.
5. Optional sweetening: If you want the juice to be a little sweeter, you can add 2-3 tablespoons of honey and mix again.
6. Strain the juice: Strain the blended juice through a fine sieve or a nut milk bag to remove pulp and seeds, adding water if necessary.
7. Serve cold.

This recipe makes about 1000 ml of pomegranate apple juice, which helps protect the skin from damage caused by UV rays and pollution and is rich in vitamin C.

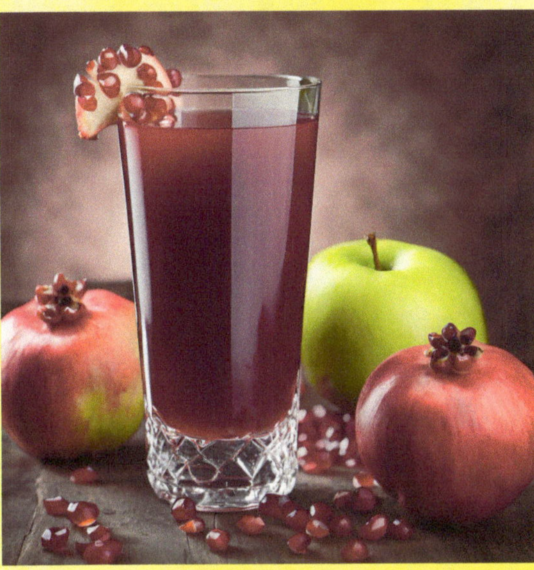

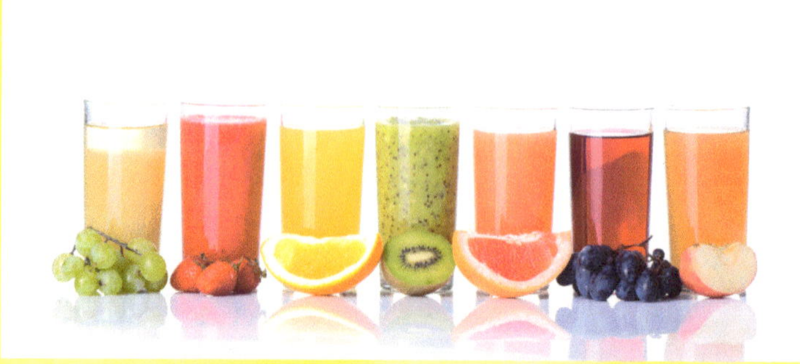

13.-18. Juices for weight loss:
Light, tasty and full of energy

The path to a healthier body weight can be delicious and refreshing – with our juices for weight loss.

These specially formulated juices contain a balanced blend of nutrient-rich ingredients such as metabolism-boosting ginger, fat-burning grapefruit, fiber-rich spinach and refreshing cucumber.

They are low in calories but full of vitamins, minerals and antioxidants that provide the body with energy while curbing appetite.

The natural ingredients support digestion, promote metabolism and help to gently detoxify the body.

Enjoy these delicious juices as part of a balanced diet plan and make losing weight a healthy, enjoyable experience.

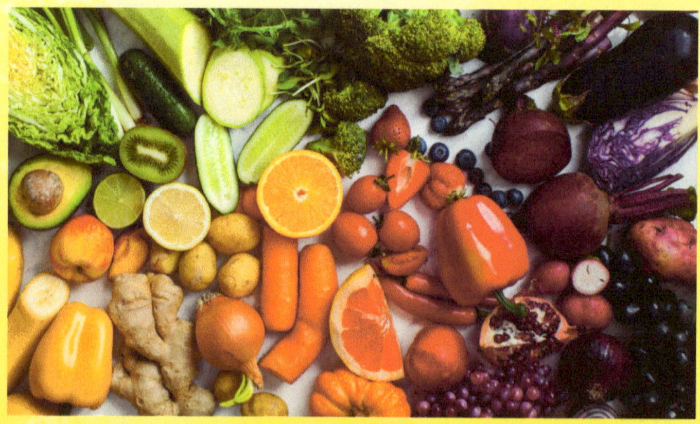

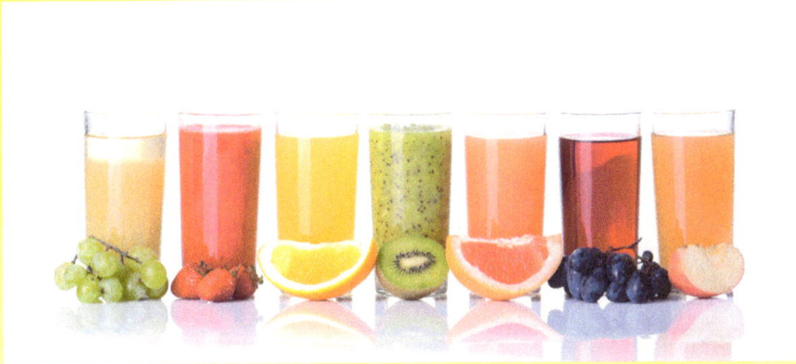

13. Grapefruit cinnamon juice (1000 ml)

Ingredients:
- 2 large grapefruits (approx. 400 ml juice)
- 4 medium-sized apples (preferably Granny Smith, approx. 500 ml juice)
- 1 small carrot
- 1/2 lemon
- 1 teaspoon ground cinnamon**
- 2 cm fresh ginger** (peeled and finely grated)
- 100 ml water
- Honey or sugar substitute to taste

Preparation:
1. Juice the grapefruit: Halve the grapefruits and squeeze out the juice. Squeeze the lemon. You should get about 400 ml of juice.
2. Juice the apples: Wash the apples, core them and cut them into pieces. Clean the carrot and chop it into small pieces.
Then process in a juicer to juice about 500 ml.
3. Add ginger and cinnamon: Add the freshly grated ginger and ground cinnamon to the juice and stir well until the cinnamon is evenly distributed.
4. Add honey or sugar substitute to taste.
5. Optionally top up with water, depending on the desired intensity of the taste.
6. Serve cold.

This recipe makes about 1000 ml of pomegranate-apple juice, which promotes fat burning and boosts the metabolism.

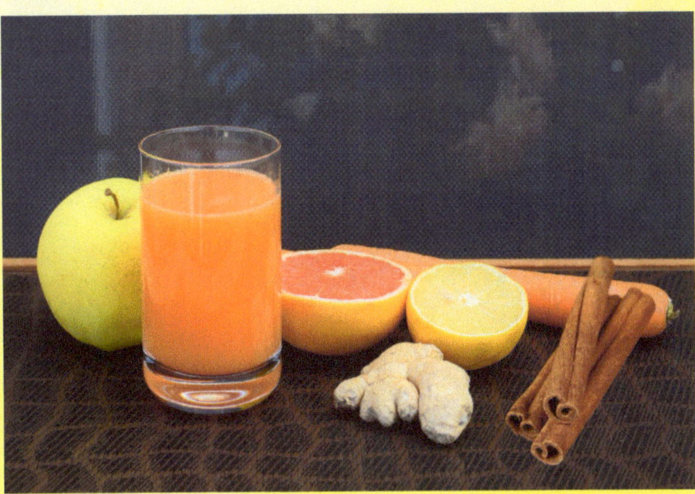

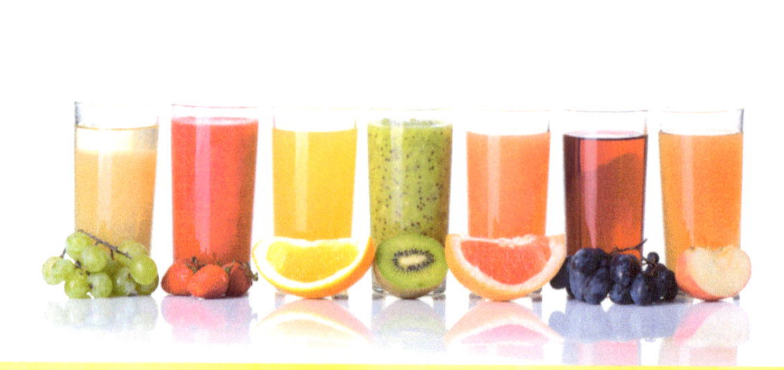

14. Pineapple spinach juice (1000 ml)

Ingredients:
- 1/2 large pineapple (approx. 350-400 g pulp)
- 2 handfuls of fresh spinach (approx. 100 g)
- 1/2 cucumber (approx. 150 g)
- Juice of 1 lemon
- 200-300 ml water
- 1-2 teaspoons honey, to taste

Preparation:
1. Prepare the pineapple: Peel the pineapple, remove the hard core and cut the pulp into pieces. You should get about 350-400 g of pulp.
2. Wash the spinach: Wash the fresh spinach thoroughly and drain.
3. Prepare the cucumber: Wash the cucumber and cut into pieces. You can leave the peel on as it contains many nutrients.
4. Blend everything: Put the pineapple pieces, spinach, cucumber and lemon juice in a blender. Mix everything well until you reach a uniform consistency.
5. Add water: Add the water little by little until you reach a volume of 1000 ml. If the juice is too thick, you can add a little more water.
6. Add 1-2 teaspoons of honey and mix well again.
7. Serve cold.

This recipe makes about 1000 ml of pineapple and spinach juice, which is low in calories but filling, while also being rich in vitamins and minerals.

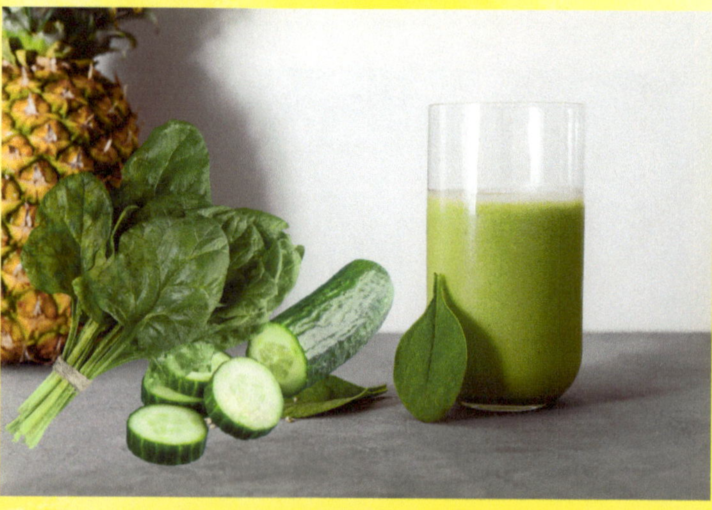

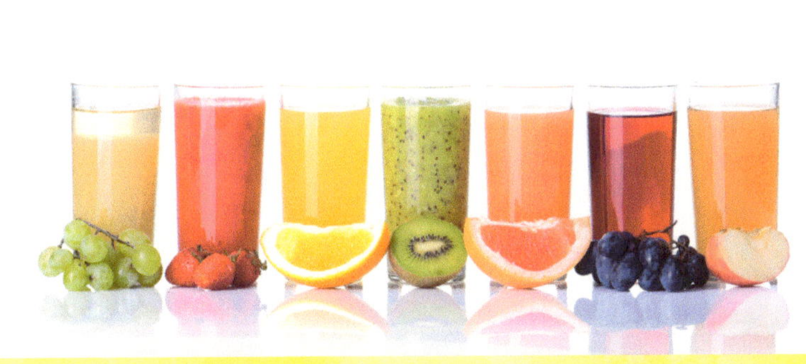

15. Watermelon mint juice (1000 ml)

Ingredients:
- 800 g watermelon pulp (without seeds)
- 1 large green apple (approx. 200 g)
- Juice of 1 lime
- 10-12 fresh mint leaves
- 1-2 tsp honey, as desired
- 50-100 ml water (depending on the desired consistency)

Preparation:
1. Peel the watermelon and cut the pulp into pieces. You should get about 800 g of pulp. The seeds should be removed as they are difficult to blend.
2. Wash the green apple, remove the core and cut into pieces.
3. Put the mint leaves in a blender together with the lime juice.
4. Put the watermelon, apple pieces, mint and lime juice in the blender. Blend everything well until a uniform consistency is achieved.
5. Sweeten the juice with honey or sugar substitute as desired.
6. If the juice is too thick, you can add 50-100 ml of water to achieve the desired consistency.
7. Serve cold.

This recipe makes about 1000 ml of watermelon mint juice, which is extremely low in calories but at the same time provides the body with fluids, vitamins and nutrients.

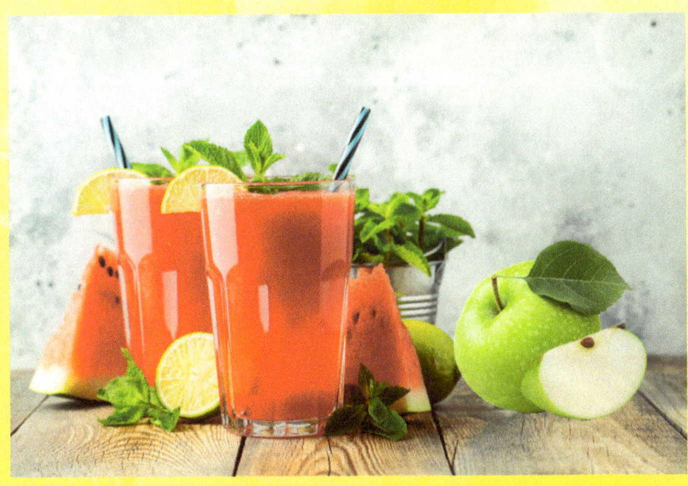

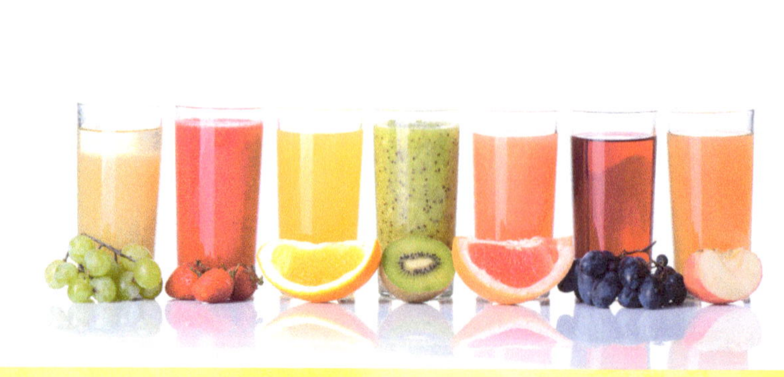

Celery-cucumber juice (1000 ml)

Ingredients:
- 6 Selleriestangen (ca. 300 g)
- 1 large cucumber (approx. 300 g)
- Juice of 1 lemon
- 2 cm fresh ginger (peeled and finely grated)
- Optional: 100-200 ml water (depending on desired consistency)

Preparation:
1. Wash the celery sticks and cut into smaller pieces.
2. Wash the cucumber and cut it into pieces. The peel can stay on as it contains many nutrients.
3. Squeeze the juice from the lemon and put it in the blender together with the grated ginger.
4. Add celery, cucumber pieces, lemon juice and ginger to the blender and mix well until a smooth consistency is achieved.
5. Optionally add water: If the juice is too thick, you can add 100-200 ml of water to reach the desired consistency.
6. Serve cold

This recipe yields about 1000 ml of celery-cucumber juice, which helps to hydrate the body,
flush out toxins and stimulate the metabolism.

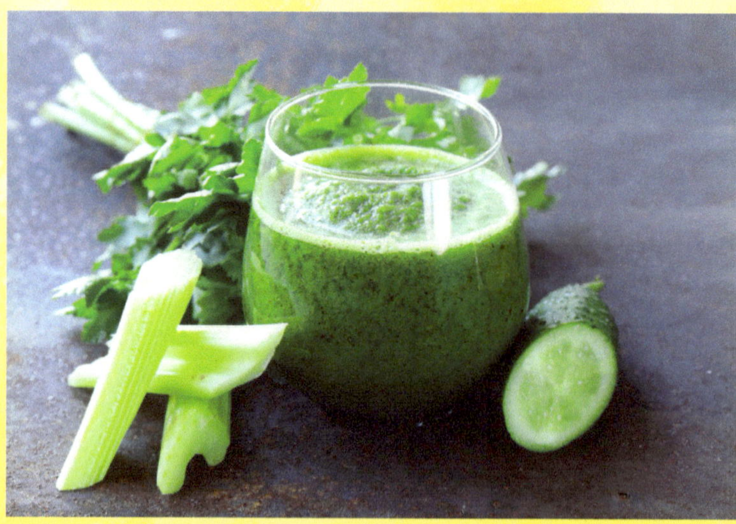

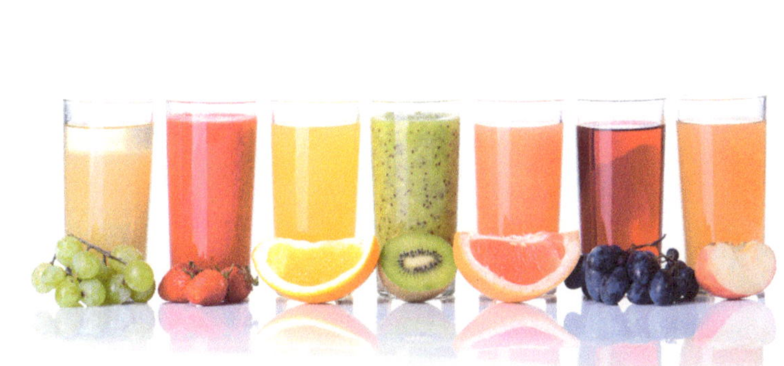

Zucchini-lime juice (1000 ml)

Ingredients:
- 2 medium-sized zucchinis (approx. 400 g)
- 1 large green apple (approx. 200 g)
- Juice of 2 limes
- 10-12 fresh mint leaves
- Optional: 150-200 ml water (depending on desired consistency)

Preparation:
1. Wash the zucchinis and cut them into pieces. You can leave the skin on as it contains many nutrients.
2. Wash the green apple, remove the core and cut into pieces.
3. Put the mint leaves and lime juice into the blender.
4. Add zucchini, apple pieces, mint and lime juice to the blender and mix well until a smooth consistency is achieved.
5. If the juice is too thick, you can add 150-200 ml of water to reach the desired consistency.
6. Serve cold.

This recipe makes about 1000 ml of zucchini-lime juice, which is filling while also providing fiber and vitamin C.

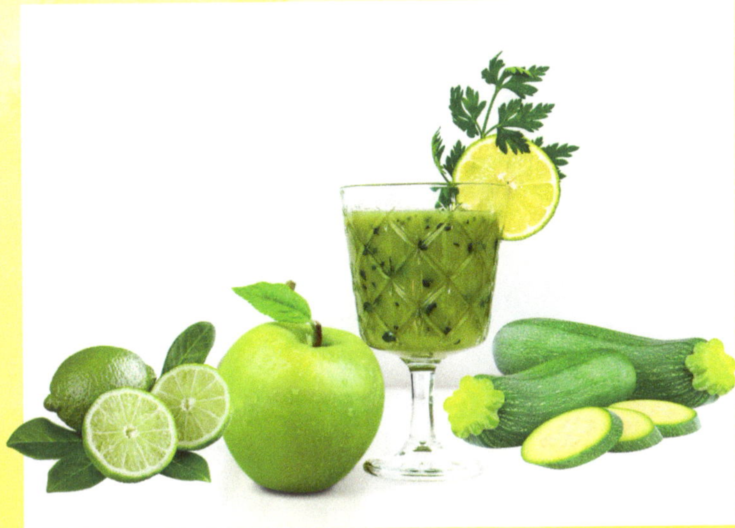

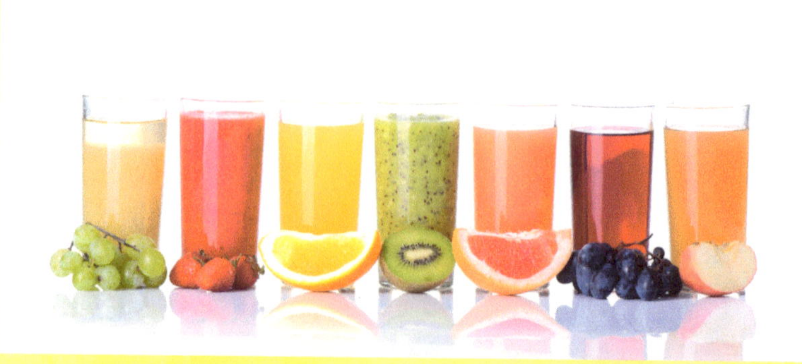

Apple-kale juice (1000 ml)

Ingredients:
- 2 handfuls of kale (approx. 100 g)
- 2 large apples (approx. 300 g, preferably Granny Smith)
- 1/2 cucumber (approx. 150 g)
- Juice of 1 lemon
- 200-300 ml water (depending on the desired consistency)

Preparation:
1. Wash the kale thoroughly and remove the hard stems. Roughly chop the leaves.
2. Wash the apples, remove the cores and cut into pieces. The peel can stay on as it contains many nutrients.
3. Wash the cucumber and cut into pieces.
4. Squeeze the juice from the lemon and put it in the blender.
5. Put the kale, apple pieces, cucumber and lemon juice into the blender. Blend everything well until you reach a smooth consistency.
6. Gradually add the water until you reach 1000 ml. If the juice is too thick, you can add a little more water.
7. Serve cold

This recipe makes about 1000 ml of apple kale juice, which is rich in vitamins, minerals and antioxidants.

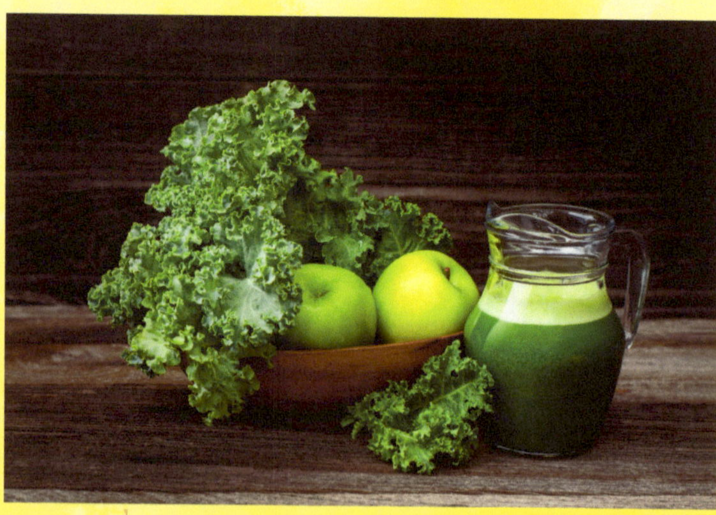

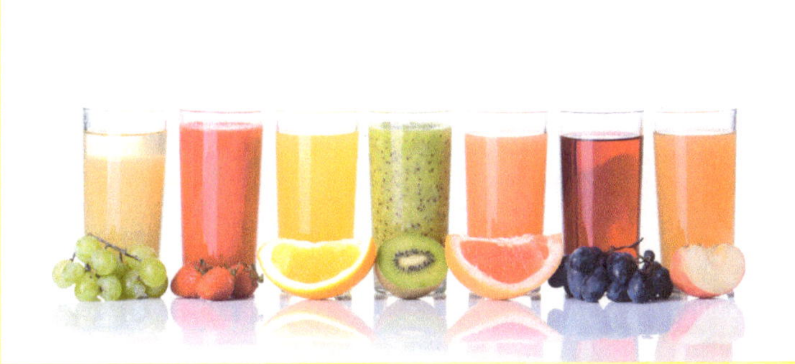

19.-24. Liver cleansing juices

Liver cleansing juices are an excellent way to support liver health and promote the body's natural detoxification.

Containing a carefully selected combination of ingredients rich in antioxidants, vitamins and minerals, these juices support liver function by providing the body with essential nutrients that help the liver process and eliminate toxins efficiently.

Regular consumption of such juices can help improve digestion, increase energy levels and strengthen the immune system. At the same time, they can help hydrate the body and promote general well-being.

As part of a balanced diet, liver cleansing juices offer a natural and tasty way to support health from the inside out and free the body of unnecessary stress.

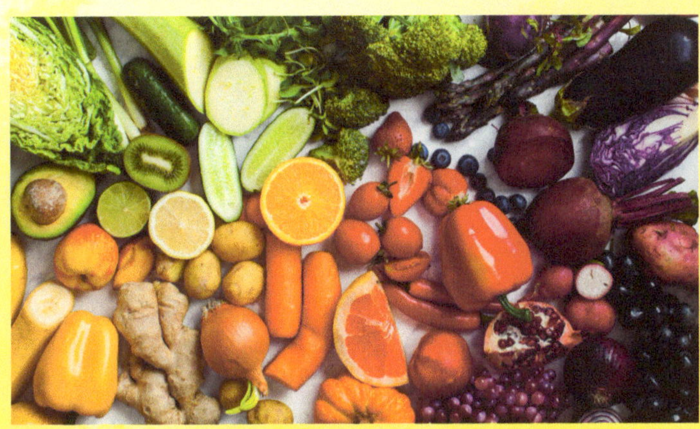

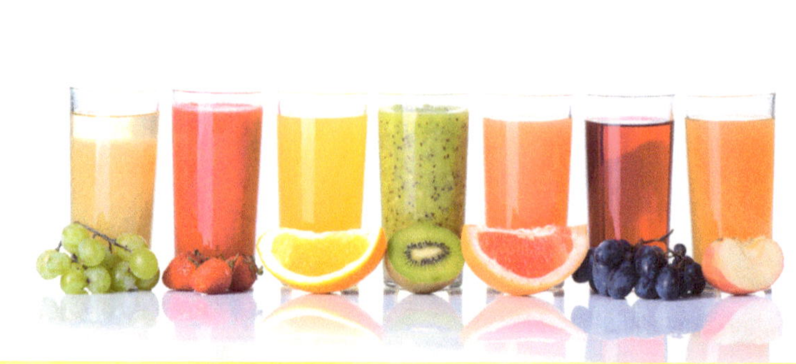

19. Beetroot-apple-lemon juice (1000 ml)

Ingredients:
- 2 medium-sized beetroots (approx. 300 g)
- 2 large apples (approx. 300 g, preferably Granny Smith)
- Juice of 1 lemon
- 2 cm fresh ginger (peeled and finely grated)
-Celery (optional)
- 300-400 ml water (depending on the desired consistency)

Preparation:
1. Peel the beetroot and cut into small pieces.
2. Wash the apples (and celery if necessary), remove the core and cut into pieces. The peel can stay on as it contains many nutrients.
3. Squeeze the juice from the lemon and put it in the blender together with the grated ginger.
4. Put the beetroot, apple pieces, lemon juice and ginger into the blender and mix well until a smooth consistency is achieved.
5. Gradually add the water until you reach 1000 ml. If the juice is too thick, you can add a little more water.
6. Serve cold

This recipe makes about 1000 ml of beetroot-apple-lemon juice, which naturally supports liver detoxification.

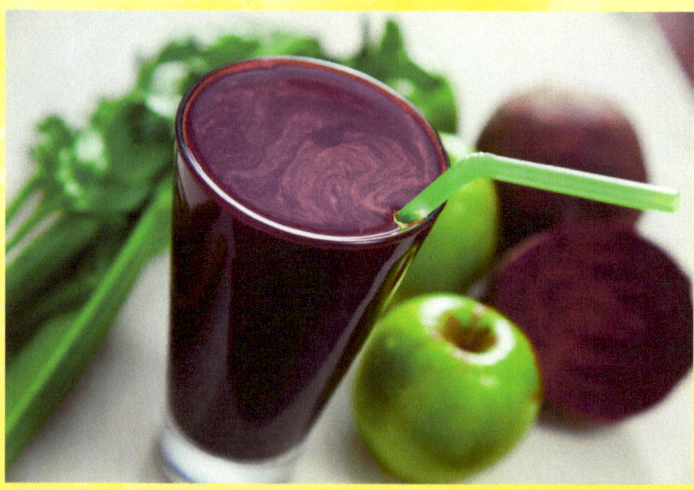

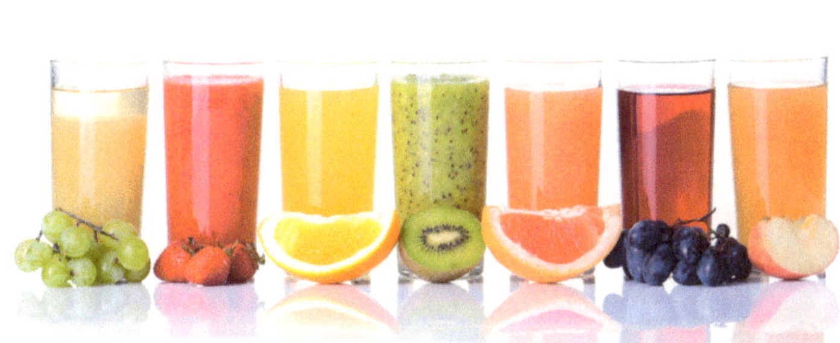

20. Dandelion-cucumber juice (1000 ml)

Ingredients:
- 2 handfuls of fresh dandelion leaves (approx. 50 g)
- 1 large cucumber (approx. 300 g)
- 2 medium-sized apples (approx. 300 g)
- Juice of 1 lemon
- 1-2 teaspoons of honey (to taste)
- 200-300 ml water (depending on the desired consistency)

Preparation:
1. Wash the fresh dandelion leaves thoroughly and let them drain.
2. Wash the cucumber and cut into pieces. Wash the apples, remove the cores and also cut into pieces.
3. Squeeze the juice from the lemon and put it in the blender together with the honey.
4. Add dandelion leaves, cucumber, apple pieces, lemon juice and honey to the blender and mix well until a smooth consistency is achieved.
5. Gradually add the water until you reach 1000 ml. If the juice is too thick, you can add a little more water.
6. Serve cold

This recipe makes about 1000 ml of dandelion-cucumber juice, which supports the liver and strengthens the liver naturally.

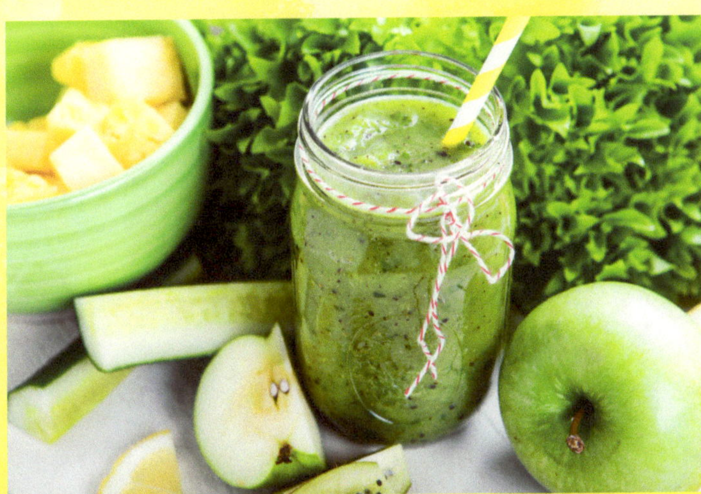

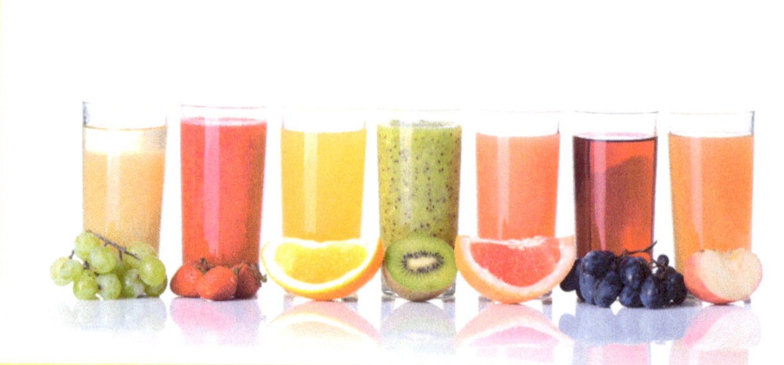

21. Turmeric-Apple-Carrot Juice (1000 ml)

Ingredients:
- 1 piece of fresh turmeric (approx. 3 cm, peeled and cut into pieces)
- 2 medium-sized apples (approx. 300 g)
-Ginger finely grated (to taste)
- 3 medium-sized carrots (approx. 300 g)
- Juice of 2 lemons
- 200-300 ml water (depending on the desired consistency)

Preparation:
1. Peel the fresh turmeric and cut into small pieces. Grate the ginger.
2. Wash the apples, remove the cores and cut into pieces. Wash the carrots, peel them and also cut them into pieces.
3. Squeeze the juice from the lemons and put it in the blender.
4. Add turmeric, ginger, apple pieces, carrots and lemon juice to the blender and mix well until a smooth consistency is achieved.
5. Gradually add the water until you reach 1000 ml. If the juice is too thick, you can add a little more water.
6. Serve cold.

This recipe makes about 1000 ml of turmeric-apple-carrot juice, which is a powerful detoxifying juice that supports liver function and provides important nutrients.

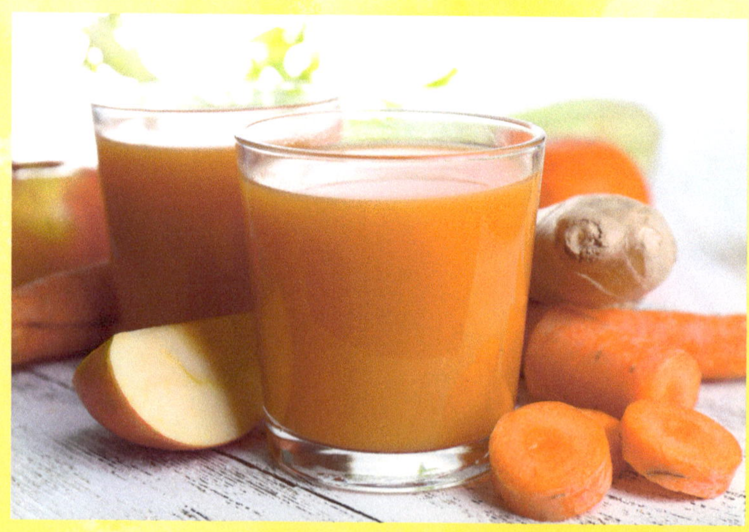

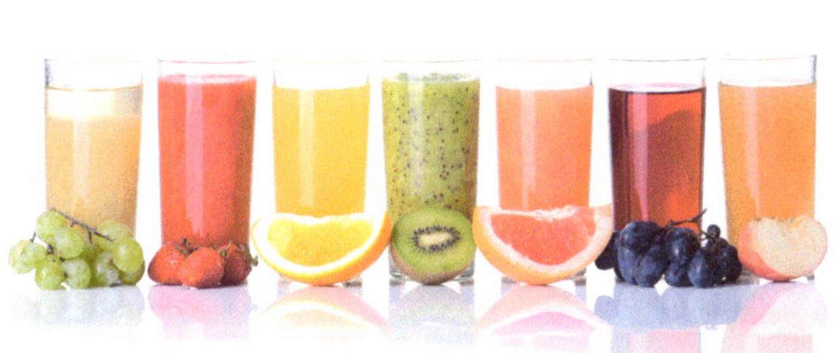

22. Artichoke-spinach juice (1000 ml)

Ingredients:
- 200 g artichoke hearts (from the jar, well drained)
- 150 g fresh spinach
- 1 cucumber (approx. 300 g)
- 1 lemon
- 300 ml water

Preparation:
1. Wash the spinach thoroughly and drain.
2. Wash the cucumber and cut into large pieces. Peel the lemon and also cut into pieces.
3. Remove artichoke hearts from the jar, drain and rinse lightly.
4. Put all ingredients (spinach, cucumber, artichoke hearts, lemon) in a blender.
5. Add 300 ml of water to improve the consistency.
6. Mix everything well until you get a smooth juice.
7. Serve cold

This recipe yields about 1000 ml of artichoke-spinach juice, which cleanses the liver and supports metabolism.

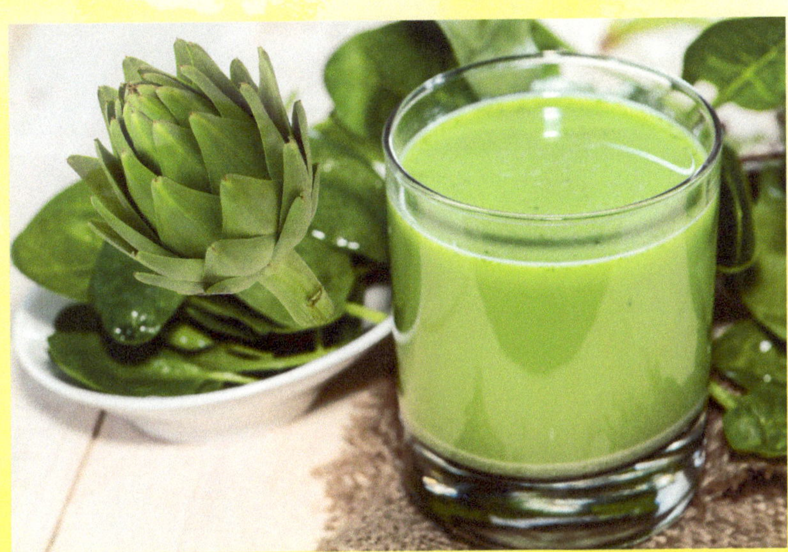

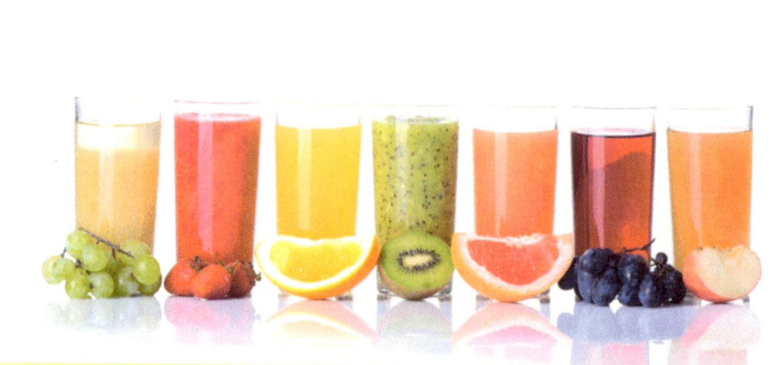

23. Radish-cucumber-apple-lemon juice (1000 ml)

Ingredients:
- 1 medium-sized radish (approx. 150 g)
- 1 cucumber (approx. 250 g)
- 2 apples (approx. 300 g)
- 1 lemon
- 200 ml water

Preparation:
1. Wash the radish and cut off the ends. Then cut into small pieces.
2. Wash the cucumber and cut into slices.
3. Wash apples, core and cut into quarters.
4. Halve the lemon and squeeze out the juice.
5. Put the radish, cucumber, apples and lemon juice into a blender along with the water.
6. Mix until a uniform consistency is achieved.
7. Serve cold.

This recipe makes about 1000 ml of radish-cucumber-apple-lemon juice, which promotes bile flow, supports the liver, and at the same time helps detoxify and hydrate thanks to the high water content of the cucumber and the fiber of the apple.

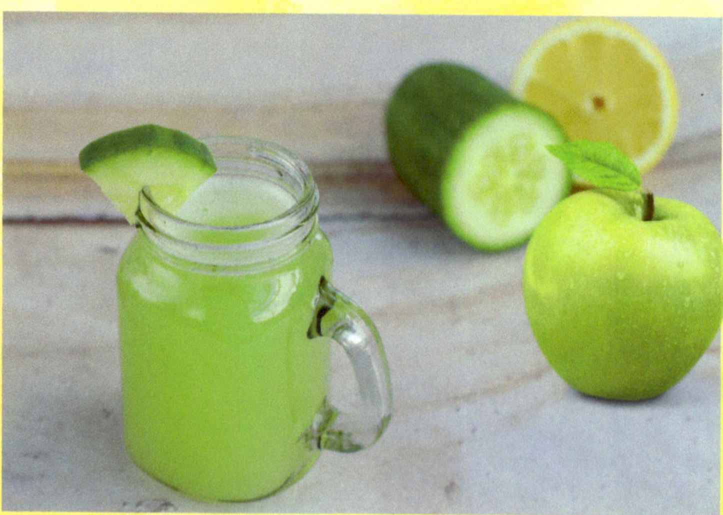

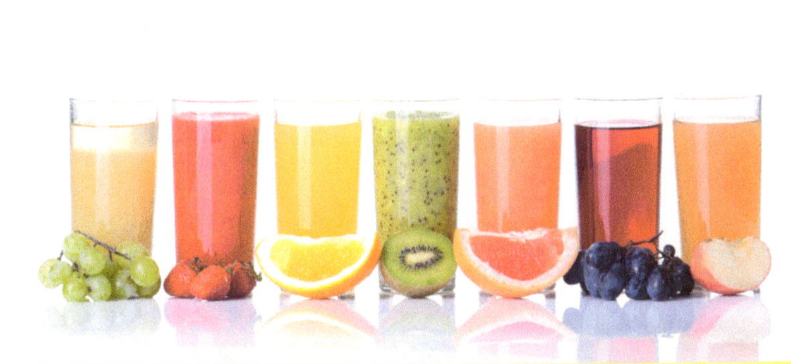

Apple-garlic-lemon juice (1000 ml)

Ingredients:
- 2 cloves of garlic
- 2 lemons
- 2 apples (approx. 300 g)
- 100 g fresh spinach
- 200 ml water

Preparation:
1. Peel the garlic and halve the cloves.
2. Halve the lemons and squeeze out the juice.
3. Wash apples, core and cut into quarters.
4. Wash the spinach thoroughly.
5. Place garlic, lemon juice, apples, spinach and water in a blender.
6. Blend until smooth.
7. Serve cold.

This recipe makes about 1000 ml of apple-garlic-lemon juice, which promotes body cleansing and supports the immune system through the powerful detoxifying properties of garlic, the antioxidant benefits of spinach and the refreshment of lemon.

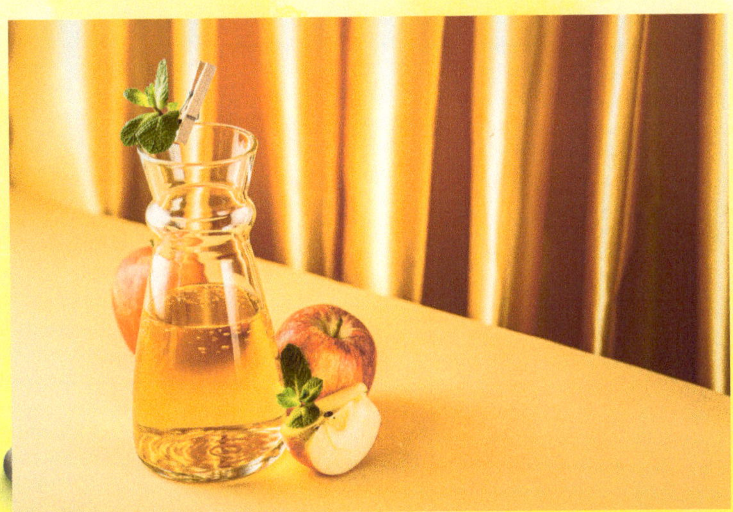

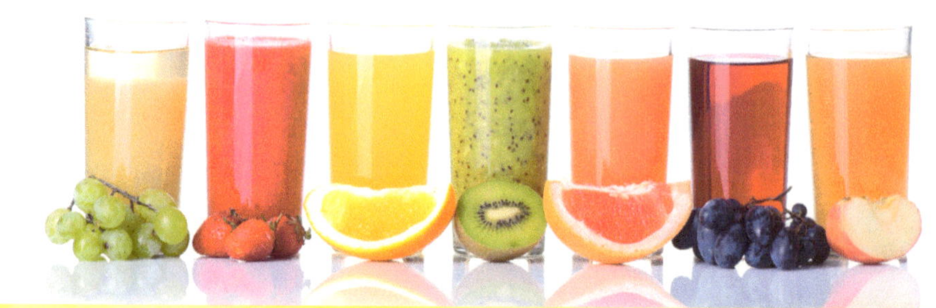

25th-30th Digestive juices

A healthy digestive tract is the key to well-being and energy - and our digestive juices are the ideal support for this.

These juices combine natural ingredients such as digestive ginger, calming peppermint, fiber-rich apples and the natural enzyme supplier pineapple to gently support digestion.

They help reduce flatulence, harmonize the intestinal flora and improve the absorption of nutrients.

Whether as a morning start to the day or as a soothing companion after a meal - these juices promote a good gut feeling and help you feel well and balanced all round.

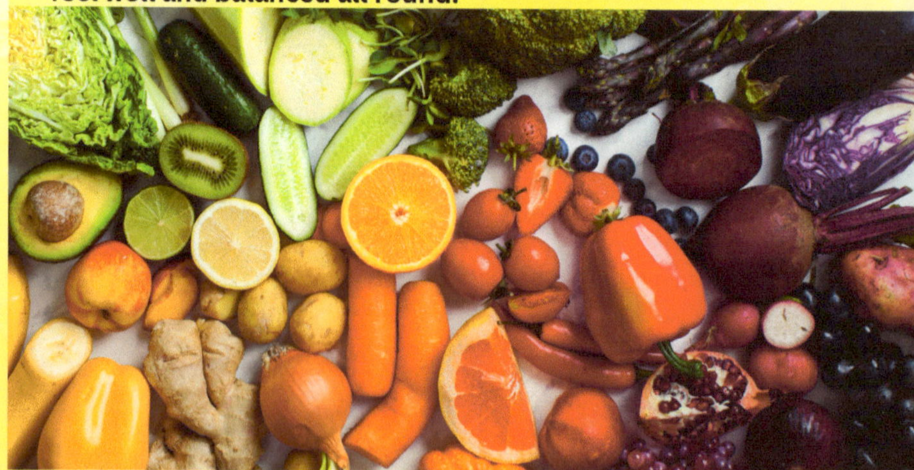

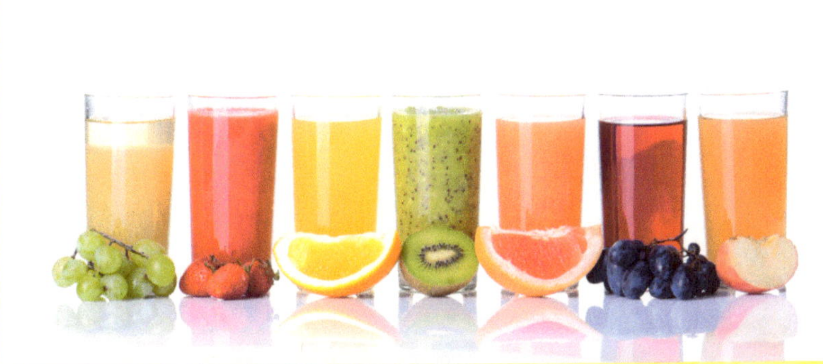

25. Apple-ginger-lemon juice (1000 ml)

Ingredients:
- 2 apples (approx. 300 g)
- 1 small piece of ginger (approx. 20 g)
- 2 lemons
- 2 Carotten (ca. 150 g)
- 2 sticks of celery
- 200 ml water

Preparation:
1. Wash apples, core and cut into quarters.
2. Peel the ginger and cut into small pieces.
3. Halve the lemons and squeeze out the juice.
4. Wash the carrots and celery, cut off the ends and cut into large pieces.
5. Place apples, ginger, lemon juice, carrots, celery and water in a blender.
6. Blend until the juice reaches a smooth consistency.
7. Serve cold.

This recipe makes about 1000 ml of apple-ginger-lemon juice, which has a soothing effect on the stomach thanks to the ginger, supports digestion and at the same time provides valuable vitamins and antioxidants thanks to the carrots and apples.

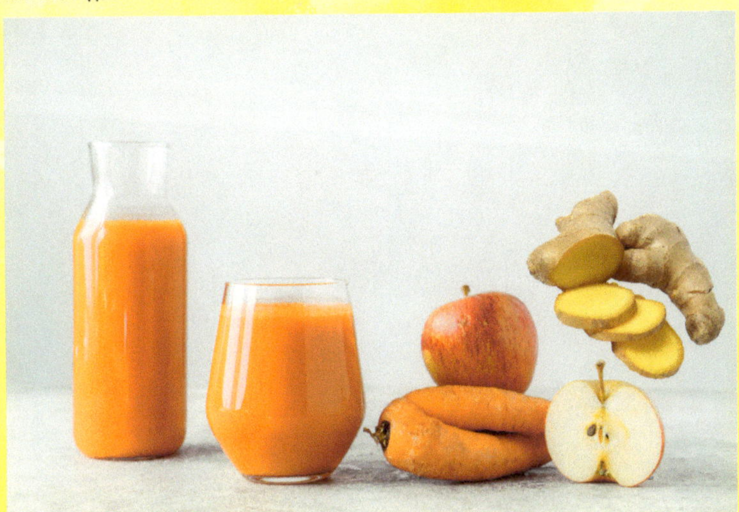

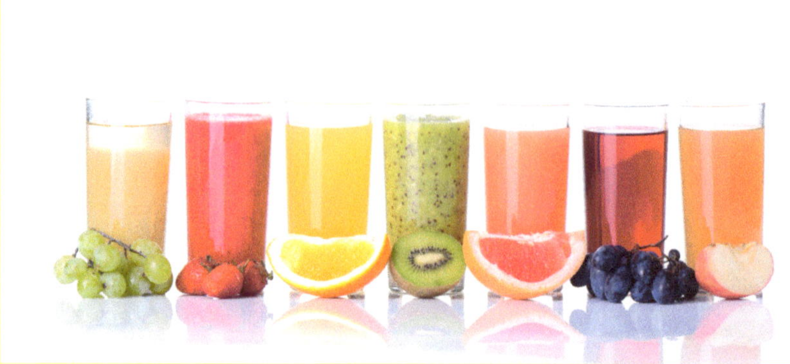

26. Fennel-apple juice (1000 ml)

Ingredients:
- 1 Fenchelknolle (ca. 200 g)
- 2 apples (approx. 300 g)
- 1 cucumber (approx. 250 g)
- 1 lemon
- 200 ml water

Preparation:
1. Wash the fennel, remove the stalk and cut into pieces.
2. Wash apples, core and cut into quarters.
3. Wash the cucumber and cut into slices.
4. Halve the lemon and squeeze out the juice.
5. Place fennel, apples, cucumber, lemon juice and water in a blender.
6. Mix until a uniform consistency is achieved.
7. Serve cold.

This recipe yields about 1000 ml of juice, which aids digestion thanks to the carminative effect of the fennel, while providing refreshing hydration thanks to the cucumber and apple.

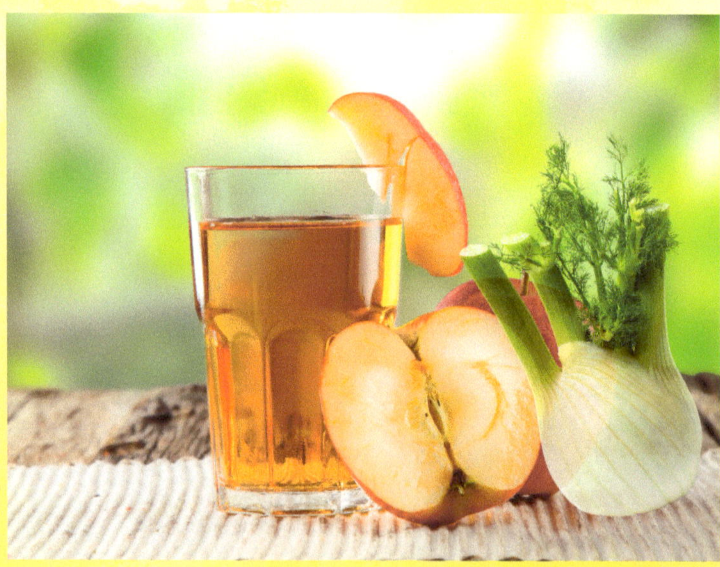

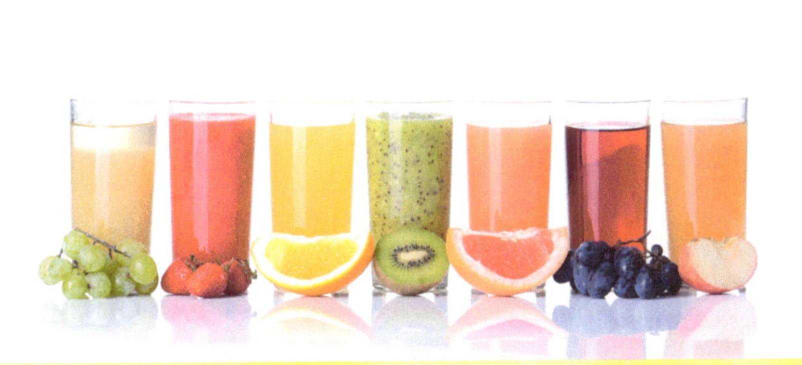

27. Papaya-mint-cucumber-lime juice (1000 ml)

Ingredients:
- 1/2 Papaya (ca. 300 g)
- 1 cucumber (approx. 250 g)
- 10 fresh mint leaves
- 2 limes
- 200 ml water

Preparation:
1. Peel the papaya, remove the seeds and cut into pieces.
2. Wash the cucumber and cut into slices.
3. Wash the mint leaves.
4. Halve the limes and squeeze out the juice.
5. Place papaya, cucumber, mint, lime juice and water in a blender.
6. Blend until the juice reaches a uniform consistency.
7. Serve cold.

This recipe makes about 1000 ml of papaya-mint-cucumber-lime juice, which aids digestion thanks to the enzymes in the papaya, while the mint and cucumber provide a refreshing effect.

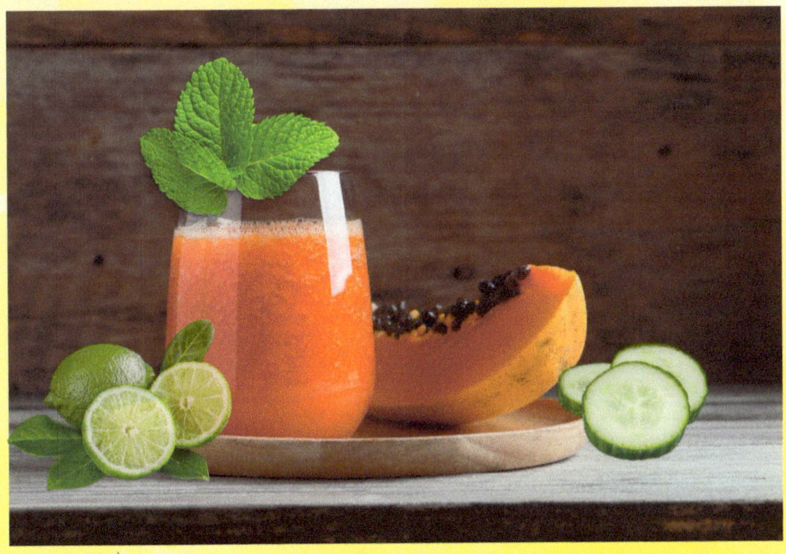

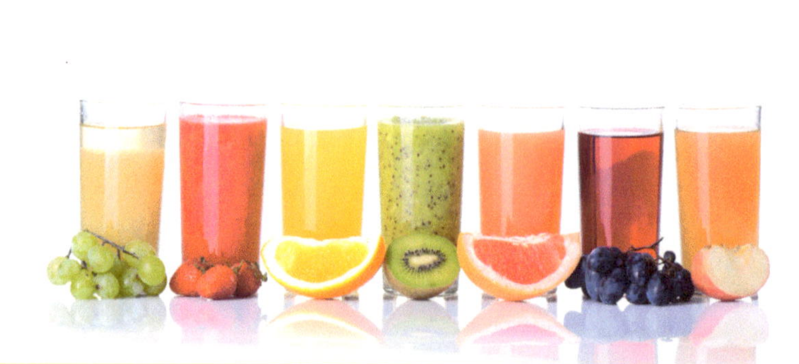

28. Carrot-fennel juice (1000 ml)

Ingredients:
- 3 Carotten (ca. 250 g)
- 1 Fenchelknolle (ca. 200 g)
- 1 apple (approx. 150 g)
- 1 lemon
- 1 tablespoon honey
- 200 ml water

Preparation:
1. Wash carrots, cut off ends and cut into pieces.
2. Wash the fennel, remove the stalk and cut into large pieces.
3. Wash the apple, core it and cut it into quarters.
4. Halve the lemon and squeeze out the juice.
5. Add carrots, fennel, apple, lemon juice and water to the blender.
6. Add honey and mix well until smooth.
7. Serve cold.

This recipe makes about 1000 ml of carrot-fennel juice, which soothes the stomach, aids digestion with the fennel and gets a slight sweetness from the honey.

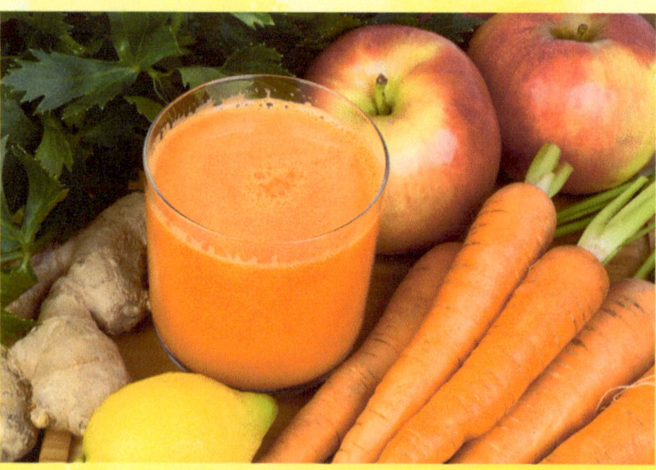

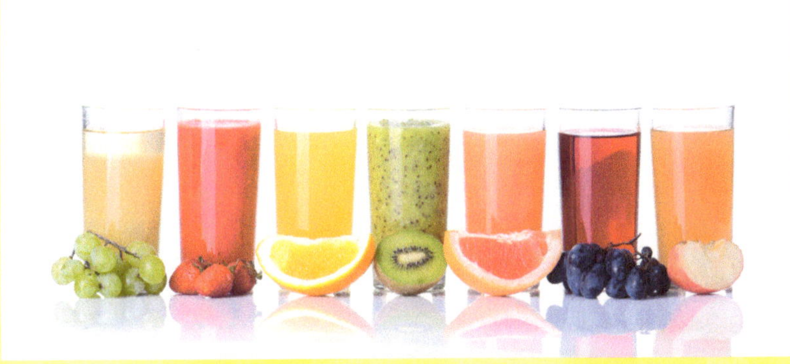

29. Pineapple-turmeric juice (1000 ml)

Ingredients:
- 1/2 pineapple (about 300 g)
- 1 teaspoon fresh turmeric (grated)
- 1 small piece of ginger (approx. 20 g)
- 1 lemon
- 200 ml water

Preparation:
1. Peel the pineapple, remove the stem and cut into pieces.
2. Peel the turmeric and grate finely.
3. Peel the ginger and cut into small pieces.
4. Halve the lemon and squeeze out the juice.
5. Add pineapple, turmeric, ginger, lemon juice and water to the blender.
6. Blend until the juice is smooth and consistent.
7. Serve cold.

This recipe makes about 1000 ml of pineapple turmeric juice, which aids digestion thanks to the bromelain in pineapple, while turmeric and ginger have anti-inflammatory effects and strengthen the immune system.

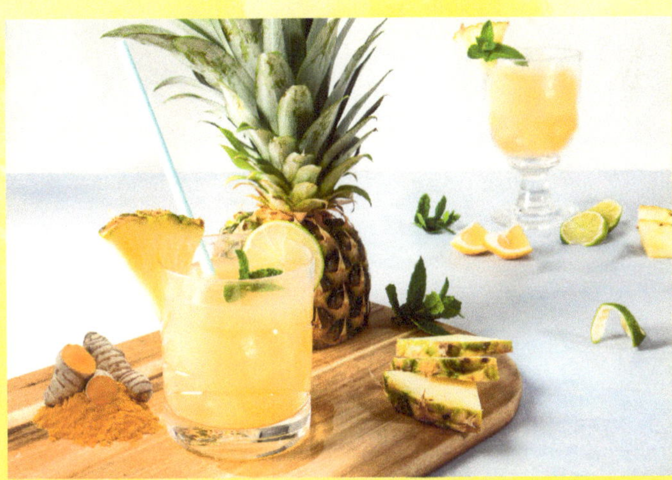

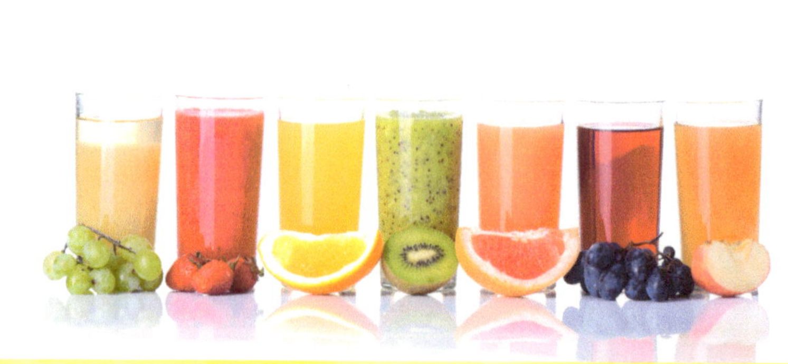

Cucumber-zucchini juice (1000 ml)

Ingredients:
- 1 cucumber (approx. 250 g)
- 1 courgette (approx. 200 g)
- 2 sticks of celery (approx. 100 g)
- 10 fresh mint leaves
- 200 ml water

Preparation:
1. Wash the cucumber and cut into slices.
2. Wash the zucchini and cut into pieces.
3. Wash the celery and cut into small pieces.
4. Wash the mint leaves.
5. Add cucumber, zucchini, celery, mint and water to the blender.
6. Mix until a uniform consistency is achieved.
7. Serve cold.

This recipe makes about 1000 ml of cucumber-zucchini juice, which is light and refreshing, aids digestion and has a cooling effect thanks to the mint.

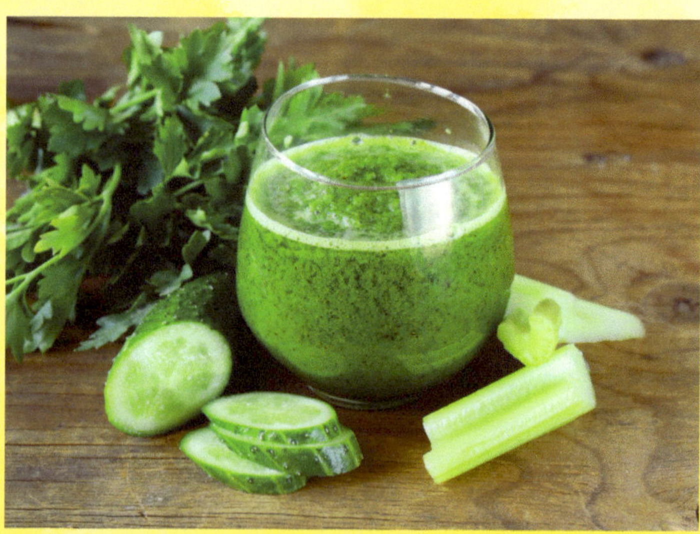

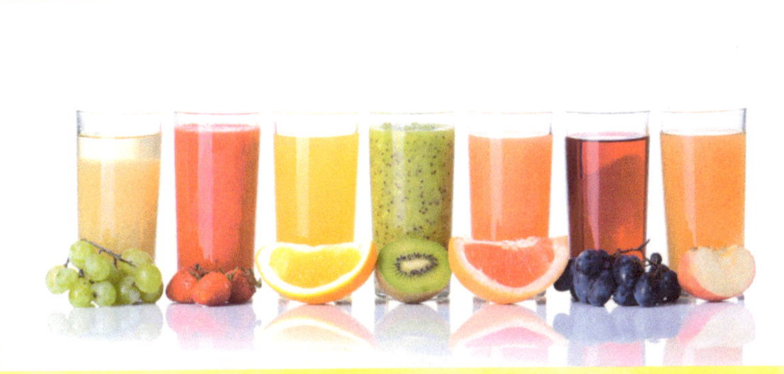

31.-36. Anti-inflammatory juices

Fight inflammation in the most delicious way – with our anti-inflammatory juices.

Rich in powerful natural ingredients like turmeric, ginger, leafy greens and vitamin-rich berries, known to have anti-inflammatory properties, these juices help the body reduce inflammation, boost the immune system and promote overall well-being.

Whether for chronic inflammation or simply for prevention, these juices offer a tasty and effective way to protect the body and counteract inflammation naturally. Enjoy this powerful blend of nutrients and antioxidants to help you stay healthy and active.

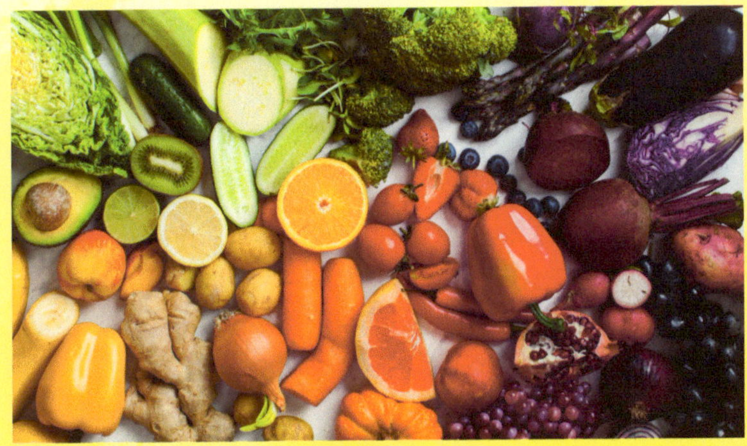

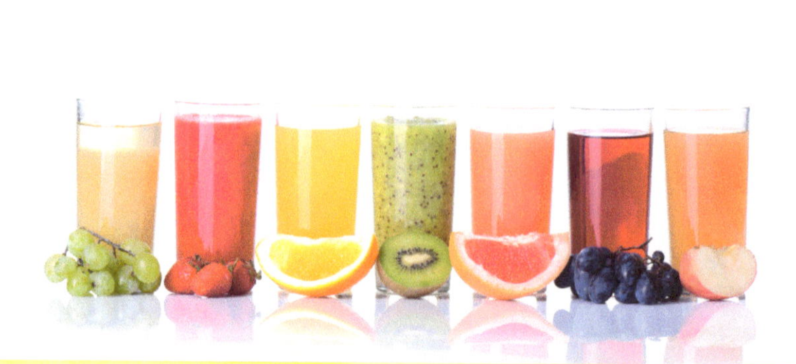

31. Turmeric-ginger juice (1000 ml)

Ingredients:
- 1 teaspoon fresh turmeric (grated)
- 1 small piece of ginger (approx. 20 g)
- 2 apples (approx. 300 g)
- 1 lemon
- 200 ml water

Preparation:
1. Peel the turmeric and grate finely.
2. Peel the ginger and cut into small pieces.
3. Wash apples, core and cut into quarters.
4. Halve the lemon and squeeze out the juice.
5. Add turmeric, ginger, apples, lemon juice and water to the blender.
6. Blend until smooth.
7. Serve cold.

This recipe makes about 1000 ml of turmeric-ginger juice, which strengthens the immune system thanks to the anti-inflammatory properties of turmeric and ginger, while also providing a refreshing effect thanks to the apple.

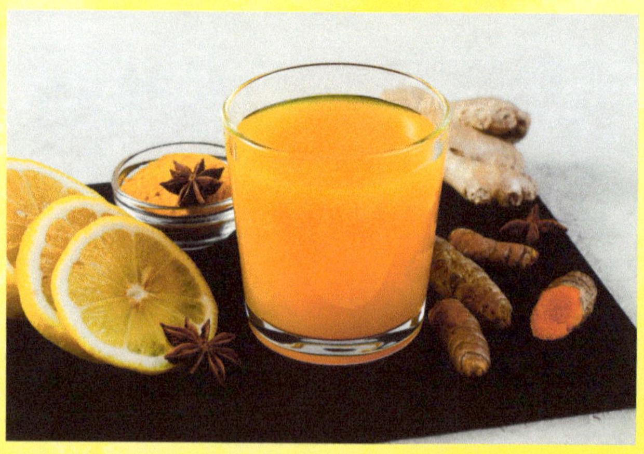

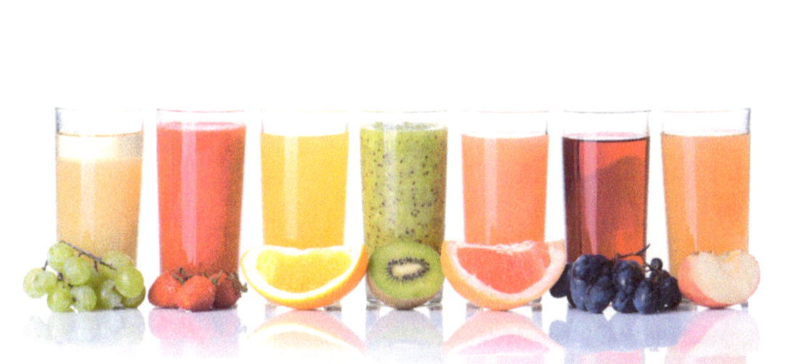

32. Blackberry-lemon juice (1000 ml)

Ingredients:
- 300 g blackberries
- 1 lemon
- 1 large apple
- 5-6 leaves of fresh mint
- 500 ml water
- 1 EL Honig (optional)

Preparation:
1. Rinse the blackberries thoroughly under cold water.
2. Halve the lemon and squeeze out the juice.
3. Wash the apple, remove the core and cut into pieces.
4. Wash the mint leaves and chop them lightly.
5. Put the blackberries, apple pieces, lemon juice and mint leaves in a blender along with the water. Add honey if desired. Blend everything well until you get a smooth juice.
6. Pour the juice through a fine sieve or cloth to remove any remaining pulp.
7. Serve cold.

This recipe makes about 1000 ml of blackberry-lemon juice, which supports cellular health and refreshes with its antioxidants.

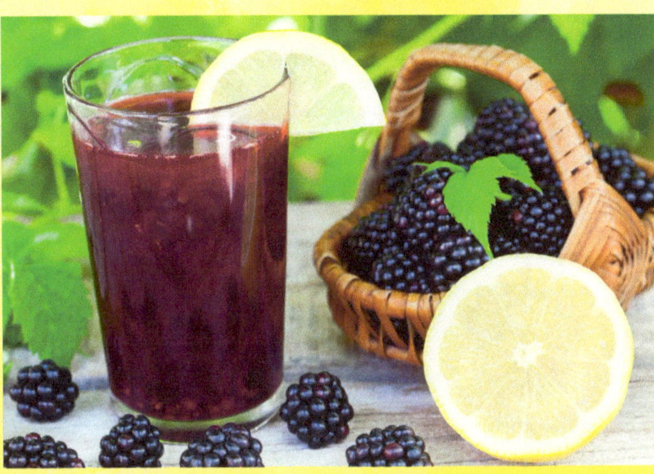

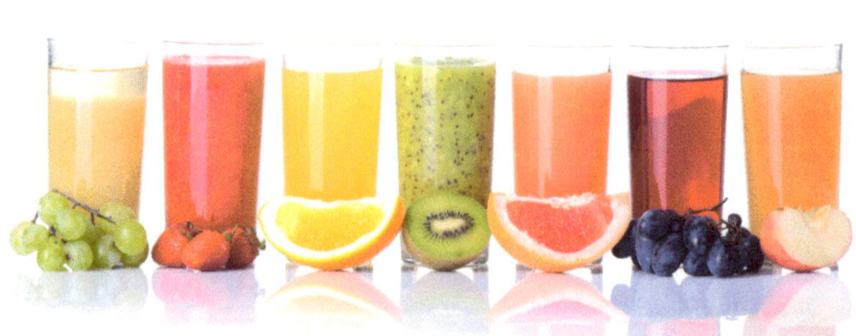

33. Mango Turmeric Juice (1000 ml)

Ingredients:
- 1 ripe mango
- 1 apple
- 1 lime
- 1 teaspoon turmeric powder (or a piece of fresh turmeric root)
- 500 ml water
- 1 EL Honig (optional)

Preparation:
1. Peel the mango, separate the flesh from the stone and cut into pieces.
2. Wash the apple, remove the core and cut into pieces.
3. Halve the lime and squeeze out the juice.
4. If using fresh turmeric root, peel it and cut it into small pieces.
5. Place mango, apple pieces, lime juice, turmeric and water in a blender.
Add honey if desired. Mix everything well until you get a smooth juice.
6. Pour the juice through a fine sieve or cloth to remove any pulp residue.
7. Serve cold.

This recipe makes about 1000 ml of mango turmeric juice, which strengthens and refreshes the immune system thanks to the anti-inflammatory properties of turmeric.

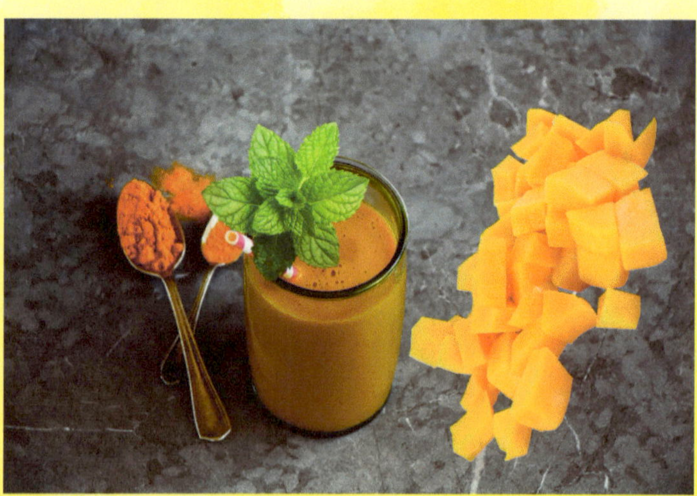

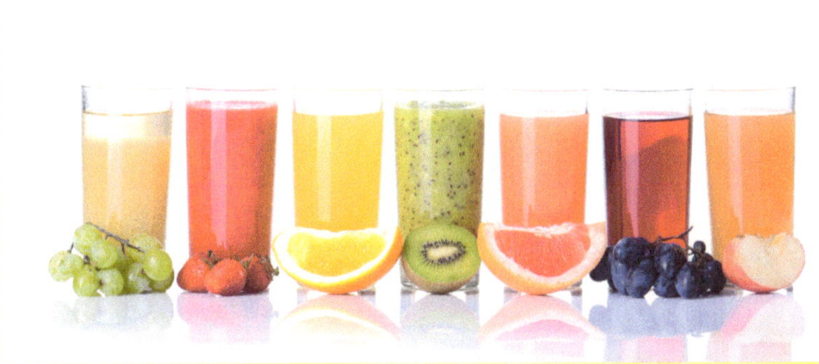

34. Pineapple-coconut juice (1000 ml)

Ingredients:
- 300 g fresh pineapple
- 200 ml coconut water
- 1 teaspoon turmeric powder (or a piece of fresh turmeric root)
- 1 lemon
- 400 ml water
- 1 EL Honig (optional)

Preparation:
1. Peel the pineapple, remove the core and cut into pieces.
2. Halve the lemon and squeeze out the juice.
3. If using fresh turmeric root, peel it and cut it into small pieces.
4. Add pineapple pieces, lemon juice, turmeric, coconut water and water to a blender.
 Optionally add the honey.
5. Mix everything well until you get a smooth juice.
6. Pour the juice through a fine sieve or cloth to remove any remaining pulp.
7. Serve cold.

This recipe makes about 1000 ml of pineapple-coconut juice, which has anti-inflammatory properties thanks to the combination of pineapple and turmeric and supplies the body with electrolytes.

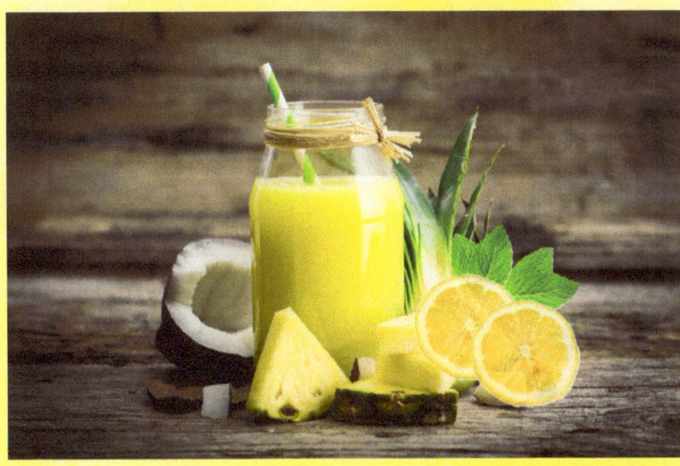

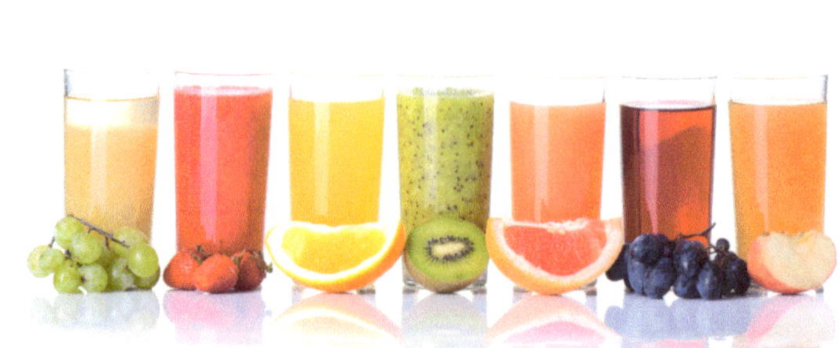

35. Spinach-cucumber-celery juice (1000 ml)

Ingredients:
- 100 g fresh spinach
- 1 cucumber
- 2 sticks of celery
- 1 small piece of ginger (approx. 2 cm)
- 400 ml water
- 1 tbsp lemon juice (optional)
- 1 TL Honig (optional)

Preparation:
1. Wash the spinach thoroughly.
2. Wash the cucumber and cut into pieces.
3. Wash the celery sticks and cut into pieces.
4. Peel the ginger and chop it finely.
5. Place spinach, cucumber, celery, ginger and water in a blender. Optionally add lemon juice and honey.
6. Mix everything well until you get a smooth juice.
7. Serve cold.

This recipe yields about 1000 ml of spinach-cucumber-celery juice, which detoxifies the body and boosts the metabolism through its cleansing effect.

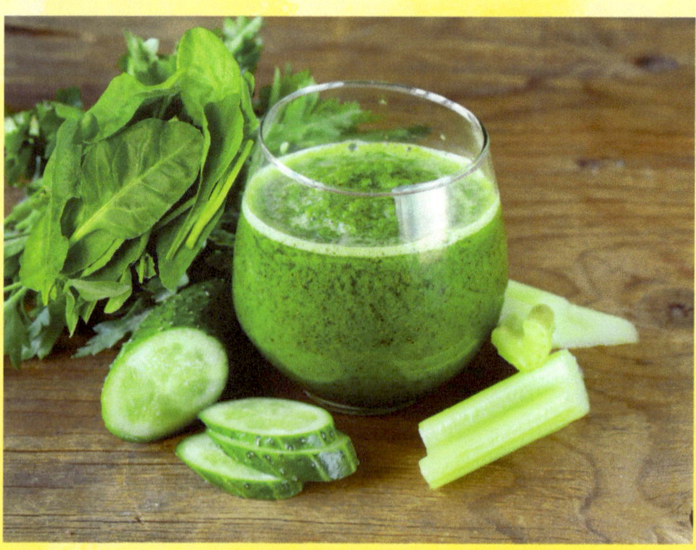

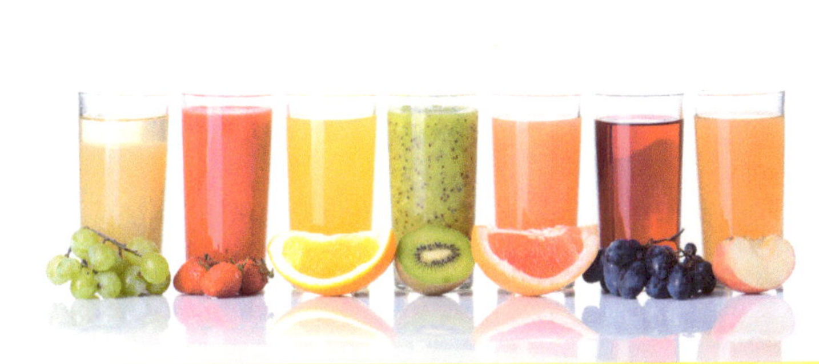

36. Beetroot-apple juice (1000 ml)

Ingredients:
- 1 medium-sized beetroot
- 2 apples
- 2 carrots
- 1 small piece of ginger (approx. 2 cm)
- 400 ml water
- 1 tbsp lemon juice (optional)

Preparation:
1. Peel the beetroot and cut into pieces.
2. Wash the apples, remove the core and cut into pieces.
3. Peel the carrots and cut them into pieces.
4. Peel the ginger and chop it finely.
5. Place beetroot, apples, carrots, ginger and water in a blender. Optionally add lemon juice.
6. Mix everything well until you get a smooth juice.
7. Pour the juice through a fine sieve or cloth to remove any solid particles. Serve cold.

This recipe makes about 1000 ml of beetroot-apple juice, which promotes blood circulation and strengthens the immune system thanks to the combination of beetroot and ginger.

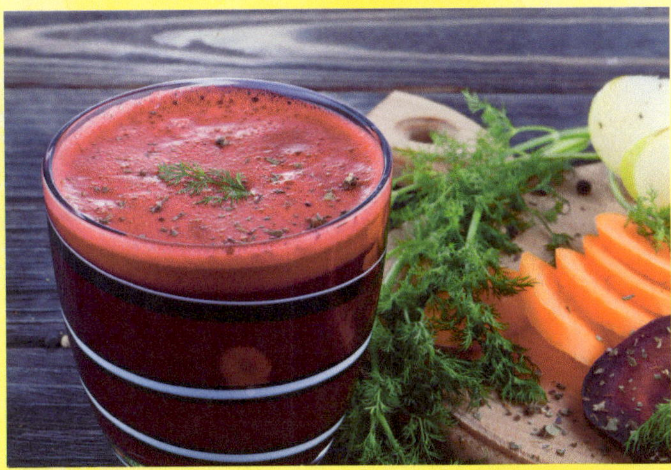

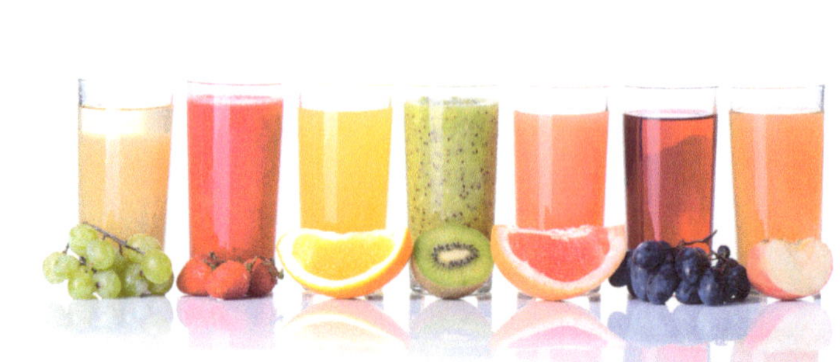

37.-42. Energy Boost-Safes

Start your day full of energy – or get a natural boost in between with our energy boost juices.

These juices are packed with invigorating ingredients like nutrient-rich spinach, vitalizing beetroot juice, refreshing apple and vitamin-rich orange.

They provide a wealth of vitamins, minerals and natural sugars that immediately supply the body with new energy and increase concentration. Whether before training, during a long day at work or as a healthy alternative to coffee - these juices give you the power you need to stay productive and focused.

Enjoy the natural energy boost that will get you through the day in a healthy way.

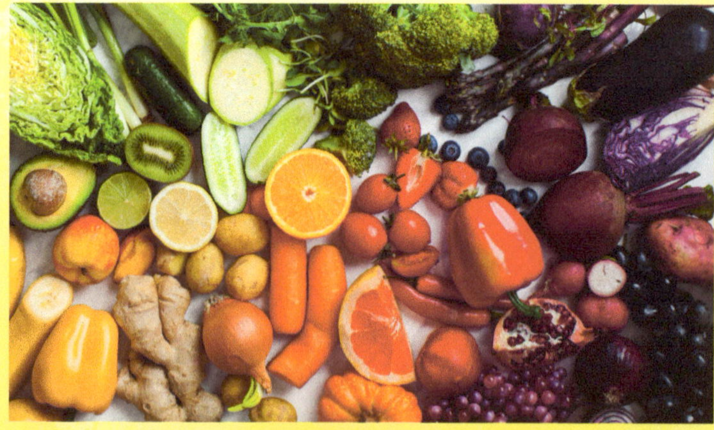

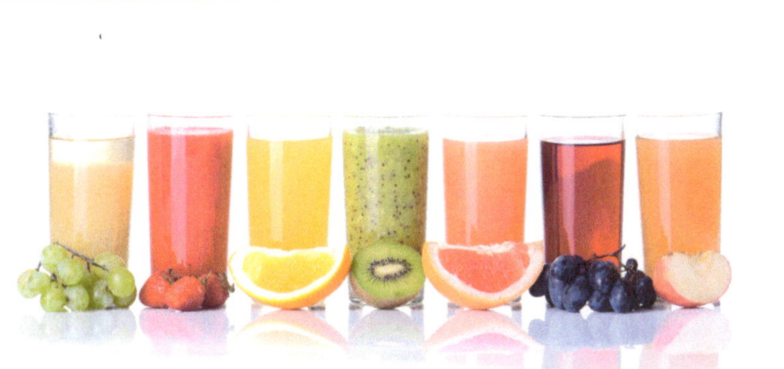

37. Orange-carrot-ginger juice (1000 ml)

Ingredients:
- 4 oranges
- 1 medium carrot
- 1 piece of ginger (approx. 3 cm)
- 1 lemon
- 250 ml water

Preparation:
1. Peel the oranges and cut them into pieces.
2. Wash the carrot thoroughly and cut into small pieces.
3. Peel the ginger and cut into thin slices.
4. Halve the lemon and squeeze out the juice.
5. Place all prepared ingredients in a blender and add the water.
6. Blend the juice on high speed until a smooth consistency is achieved.
7. Serve cold.

This recipe makes about 1000 ml of orange-carrot-ginger juice, which strengthens the immune system and invigorates with the combination of vitamin C and ginger.

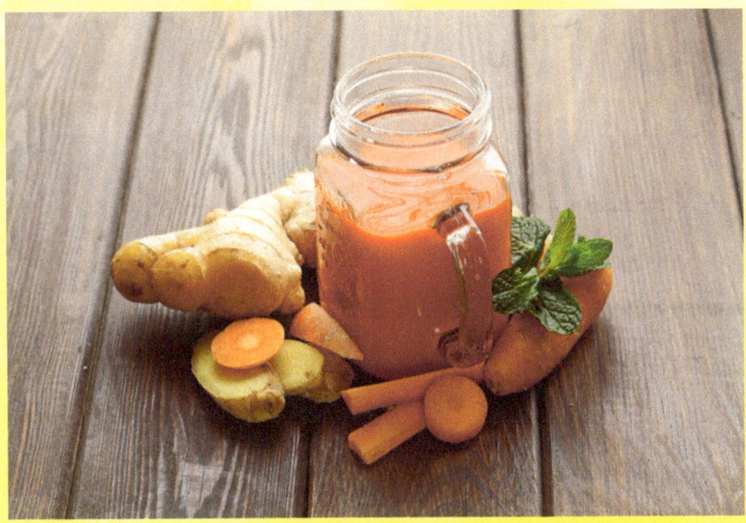

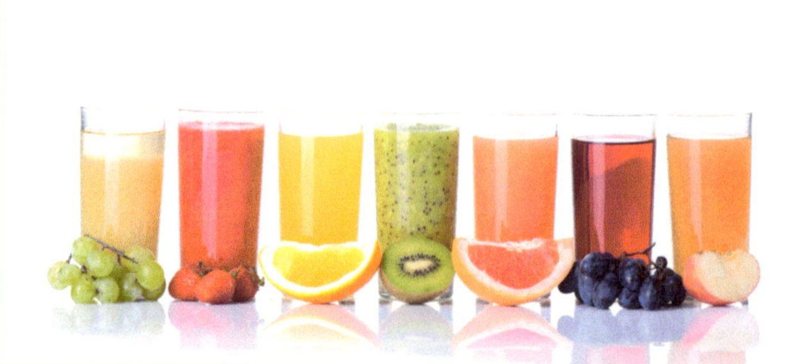

38. Apple-pear-ginger juice (1000 ml)

Ingredients:
- 3 apples
- 2 pears
- 1 piece of ginger (approx. 2 cm)
- 1 lemon
- 200 ml water

Preparation:
1. Wash the apples thoroughly, core them and cut them into pieces.
2. Wash the pears, remove the cores and cut into small pieces.
3. Peel the ginger and cut into thin slices.
4. Halve the lemon and squeeze out the juice.
5. Place apples, pears, ginger and lemon juice in a blender.
6. Add the water and mix until smooth.
7. Serve cold.

This recipe yields about 1000 ml of apple-pear-ginger juice, which tastes refreshing and pleasantly mild due to the natural sweetness of the fruit.

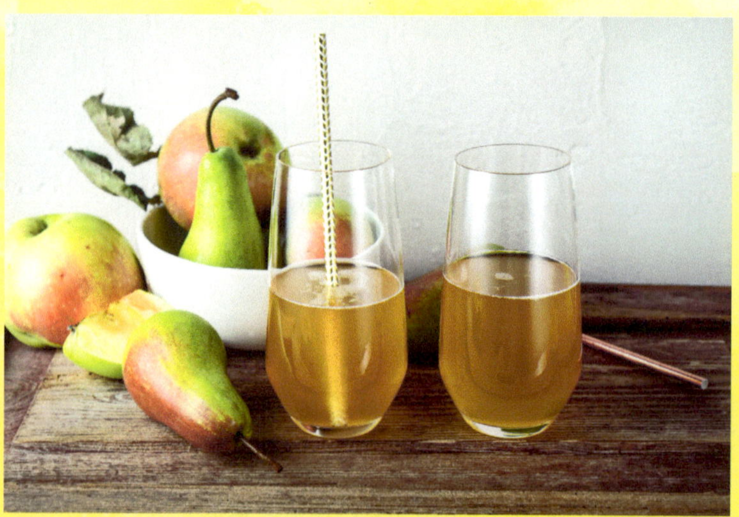

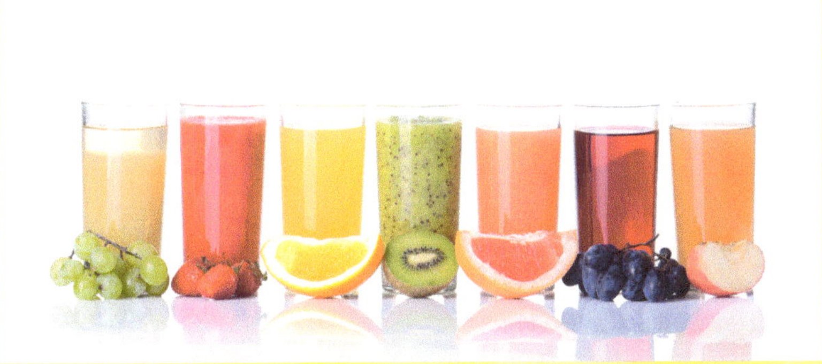

39. Grape-pomegranate juice (1000 ml)

Ingredients:
- 300 g seedless grapes
- 1 pomegranate (seeds)
- 1 apple
- 1 lemon
- 200 ml water

Preparation:
1. Wash the grapes thoroughly and remove the stems.
2. Halve the pomegranate and carefully remove the seeds.
3. Wash the apple, core it and cut it into pieces.
4. Halve the lemon and squeeze out the juice.
5. Place all ingredients, including the grapes, pomegranate seeds, apple pieces and lemon juice, in a blender.
6. Add the water and mix on high until the juice has a smooth consistency.
7. Serve cold.

This recipe makes about 1000 ml of grape-pomegranate juice, which is rich in antioxidants and strengthens the immune system.

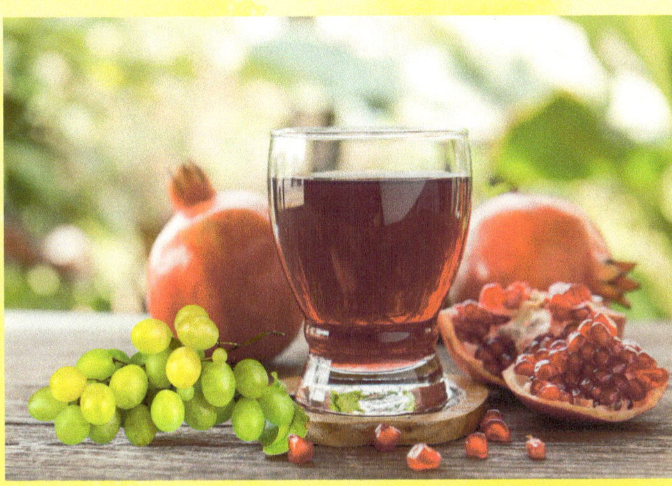

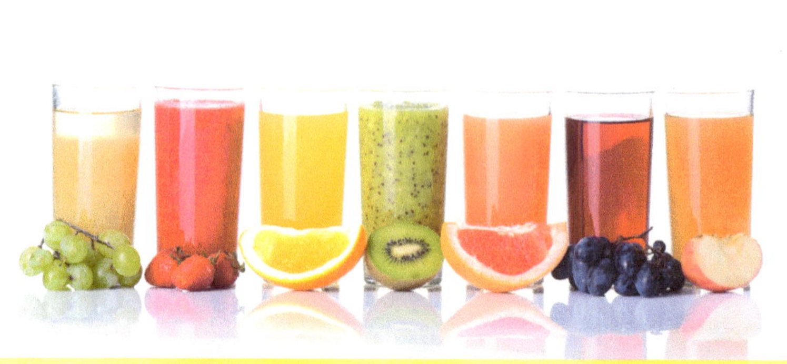

40. Spinach-Pineapple-Juice (1000 ml)

Ingredients:
- 2 handfuls of fresh spinach
- 300 g pineapple (peeled and cut into pieces)
- 1 piece of ginger (approx. 2 cm)
- 1 lime (juice)
- 250 ml water

Preparation:
1. Wash the fresh spinach thoroughly.
2. Peel the pineapple and cut it into small pieces.
3. Peel the ginger and cut into thin slices.
4. Halve the lime and squeeze out the juice.
5. Place spinach, pineapple, ginger and lime juice in a blender.
6. Add the water and mix on high until a smooth consistency is achieved.
7. Serve cold.

This recipe makes about 1000 ml of spinach-pineapple juice, which provides an energy boost thanks to the green leafy vegetables and tastes refreshing.

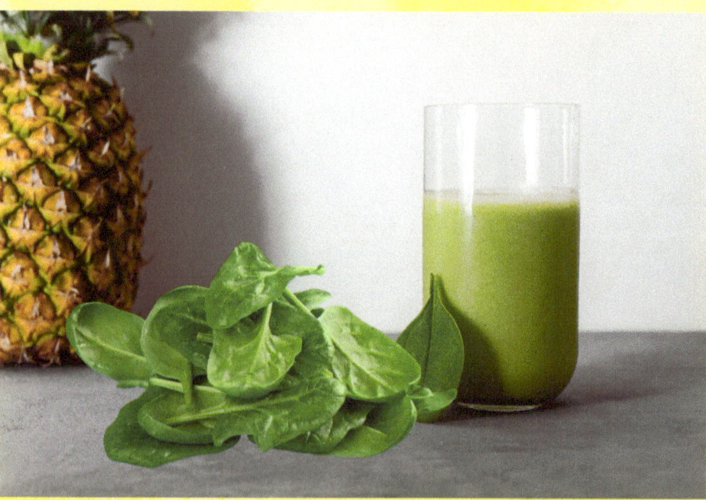

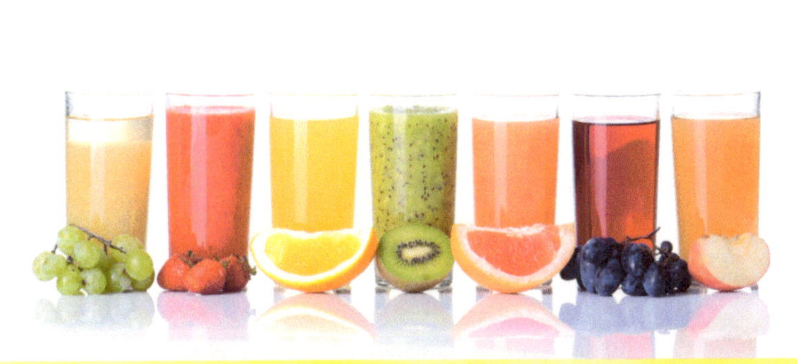

41. Apple-carrot juice (1000 ml)

Ingredients:
- 3 apples
- 2 medium carrots
- 1 stick of celery
- 1 lemon
- 200 ml water

Preparation:
1. Wash the apples thoroughly, core them and cut them into pieces.
2. Peel the carrots and cut them into small pieces.
3. Wash the celery and cut into slices.
4. Halve the lemon and squeeze out the juice.
5. Place all prepared ingredients in a blender and add the water.
6. Blend everything on the highest setting until the juice reaches a uniform consistency.
7. Serve cold.

This recipe makes about 1000 ml of apple-carrot juice, a classic that provides more energy through the combination of ingredients.

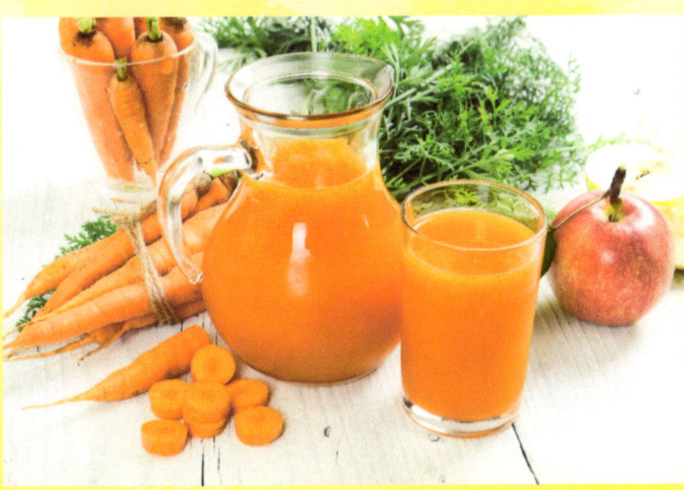

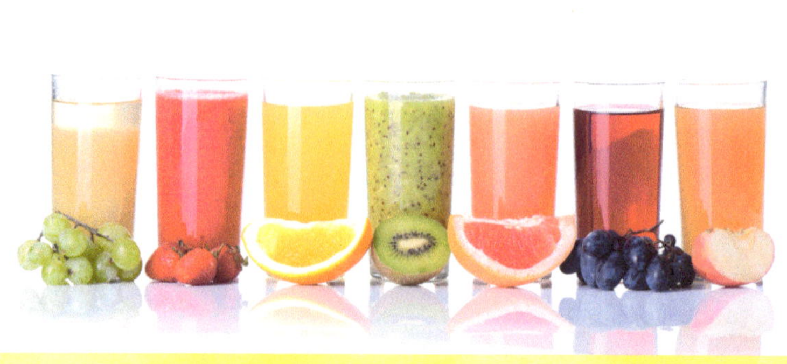

42. Beetroot and carrot juice (1000 ml)

Ingredients:
- 1 medium-sized beetroot (raw, peeled)
- 2 carrots
- 1 apple
- 1 lemon
- 200 ml water
- Honey as desired

Preparation:
1. Peel the beetroot and cut into small pieces.
2. Peel the carrots and cut them into pieces.
3. Wash the apple thoroughly, core it and cut it into pieces.
4. Halve the lemon and squeeze out the juice.
5. Place all prepared ingredients in a blender and add the water.
6. Blend everything on high speed until the juice reaches a smooth consistency.
7. Serve cold.

This recipe makes about 1000 ml of beetroot-carrot juice, which is rich in nutrients and, thanks to its invigorating effect, is ideal for an energy boost.

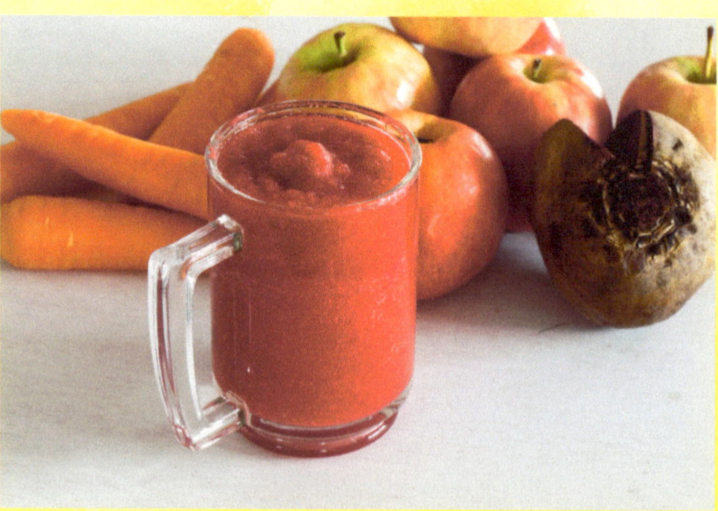

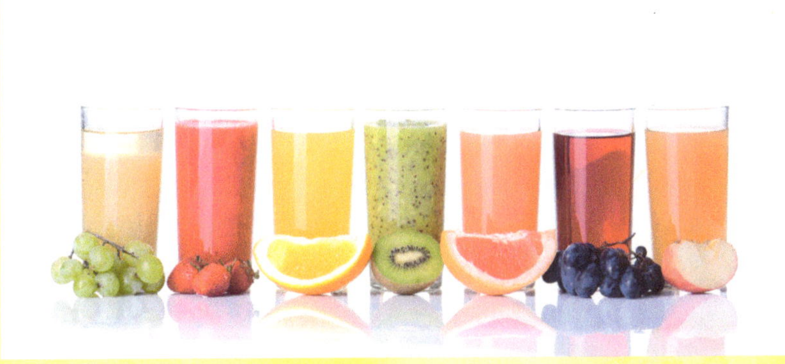

43.-48. Immune system strengthening juices

Protect yourself naturally and boost your immune system with our specially formulated juices. These juices are packed with immune-boosting ingredients like vitamin-rich citrus, antioxidant berries, anti-inflammatory ginger and immune-modulating turmeric.

They provide a high dose of vitamin C, zinc and other important nutrients known to support the immune system and protect the body against infections.

Whether for prevention during the cold season or for daily strengthening, these juices offer a delicious and effective way to support your immune system and promote your health naturally. Stay strong and healthy, sip by sip.

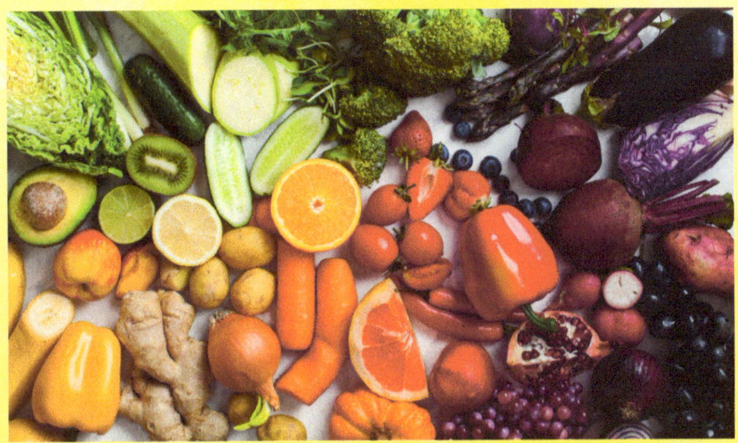

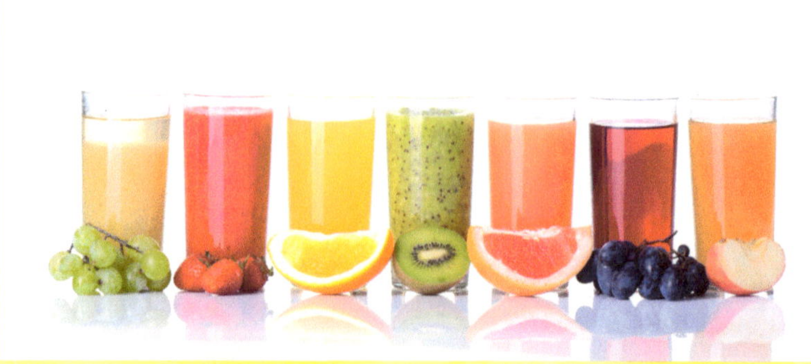

43. Lemon-Apple-Ginger Juice (1000 ml)

Ingredients:
- 3 lemons
- 1 piece of ginger (approx. 3 cm)
- 1 apple
- 2 carrots
- 200 ml water

Preparation:
1. Halve the lemons and squeeze out the juice.
2. Peel the ginger and cut into thin slices.
3. Wash the apple, core it and cut it into pieces.
4. Peel the carrots and cut them into small pieces.
5. Place lemon juice, ginger, apple pieces and carrots in a blender.
6. Add the water and mix everything on high until the juice reaches a uniform consistency.
7. Serve cold.

This recipe makes about 1000 ml of lemon-apple-ginger juice, which strengthens the immune system thanks to the vitamin C in the lemon and the ginger.

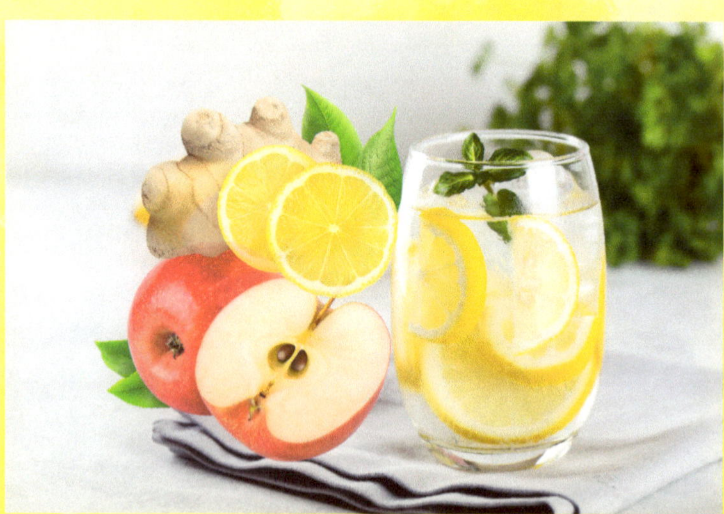

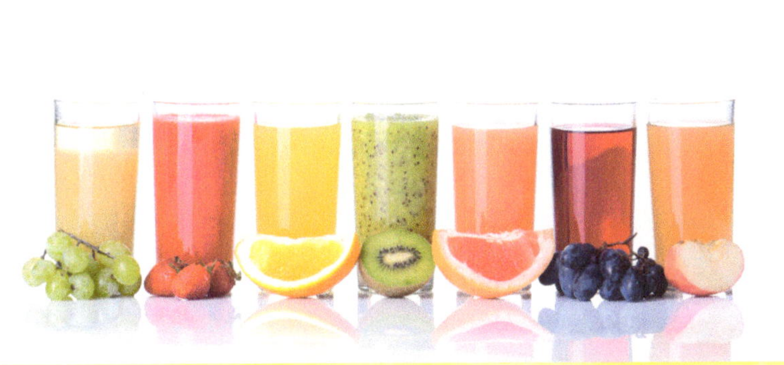

44. Orange-turmeric juice (1000 ml)

Ingredients:
- 4 oranges
- 1 piece of fresh turmeric (approx. 3 cm)
- 1 piece of ginger (approx. 2 cm)
- 1 lemon
- 200 ml water

Preparation:
1. Peel the oranges and cut them into pieces.
2. Peel the fresh turmeric and cut into thin slices.
3. Peel the ginger and also cut it into thin slices.
4. Halve the lemon and squeeze out the juice.
5. Place orange pieces, turmeric, ginger and lemon juice in a blender.
6. Add the water and mix on high until a smooth consistency is achieved.
7. Serve cold.

This recipe makes about 1000 ml of orange turmeric juice, which strengthens the immune system thanks to the powerful combination of antioxidants from turmeric, ginger and lemon.

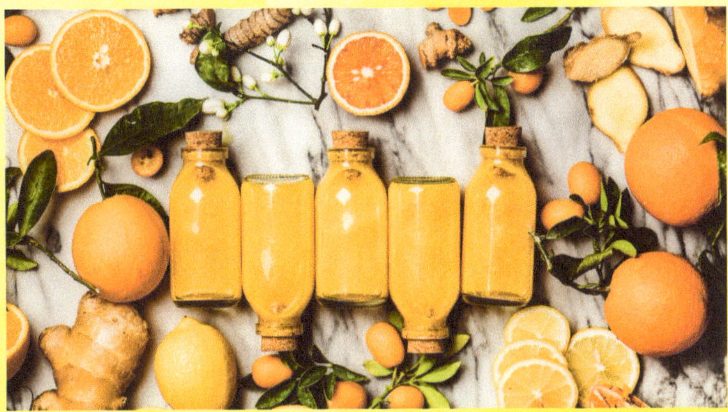

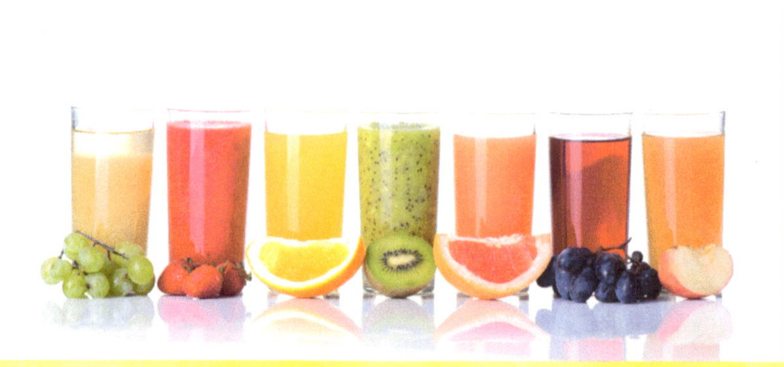

45. Mango-ginger-carrot juice (1000 ml)

Ingredients:
- 1 ripe mango
- 1 piece of ginger (approx. 2 cm)
- 2 carrots
- 1 lime (juice)
- 200 ml water

Preparation:
1. Peel the mango, remove the seeds and cut into pieces.
2. Peel the ginger and cut into thin slices.
3. Peel the carrots and cut them into small pieces.
4. Halve the lime and squeeze out the juice.
5. Place mango pieces, ginger, carrots and lime juice in a blender.
6. Add the water and blend on high until the juice reaches a smooth consistency.
7. Serve cold.

This recipe yields about 1000 ml of mango-ginger-carrot juice, which tastes sweet and strengthens the immune system with its protective ingredients.

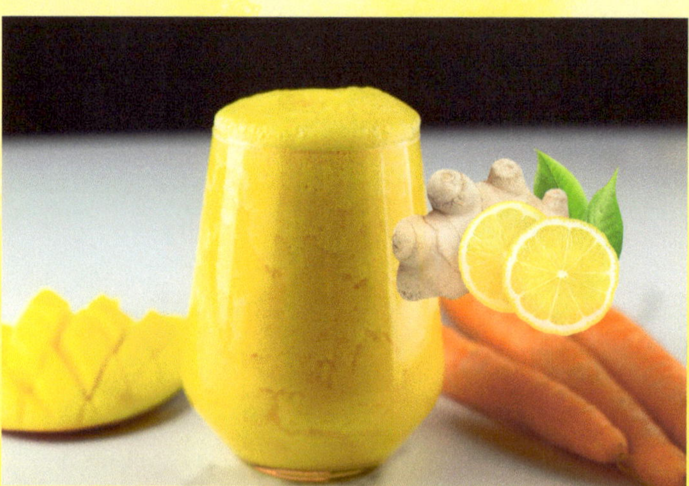

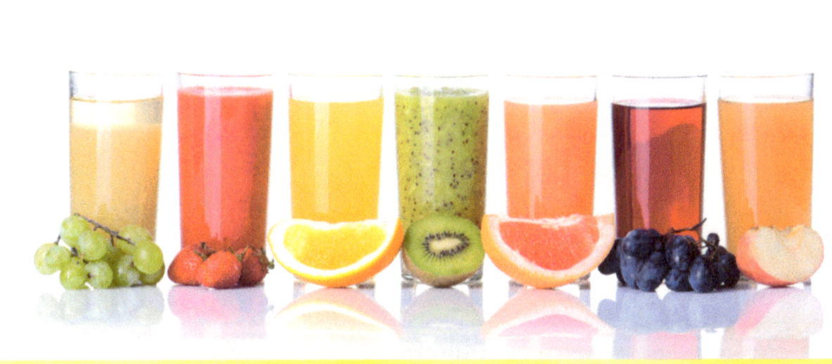

46. Kiwi-Green Tea-Apple Juice (1000 ml)

Ingredients:
- 3 Kiwis
- 1 green apple
- 1 lemon
- 200 ml cooled green tea
- 100 ml water

Preparation:
1. Peel the kiwis and cut into pieces.
2. Wash the apple thoroughly, core it and cut it into small pieces.
3. Halve the lemon and squeeze out the juice.
4. Place the cooled green tea and the prepared ingredients in a blender.
5. Add the water and mix until smooth.
6. Mix everything well until the juice is smooth.
7. Serve cold.

This recipe makes about 1000 ml of kiwi green tea apple juice, which strengthens and refreshes the immune system through the combination of kiwi and green tea.

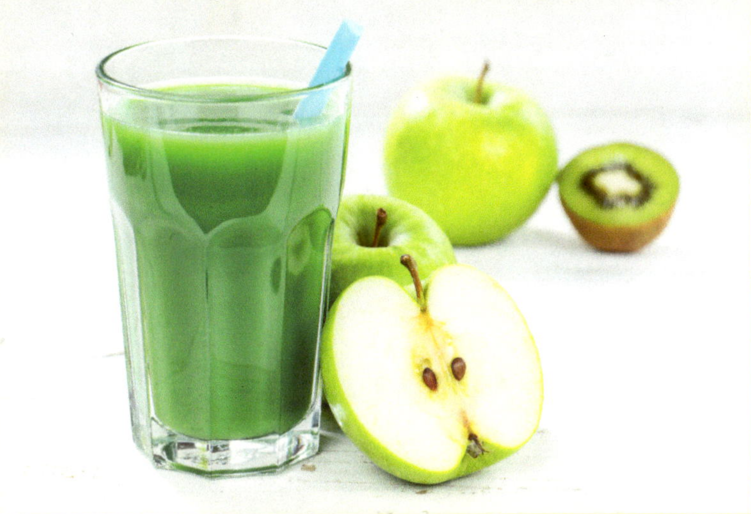

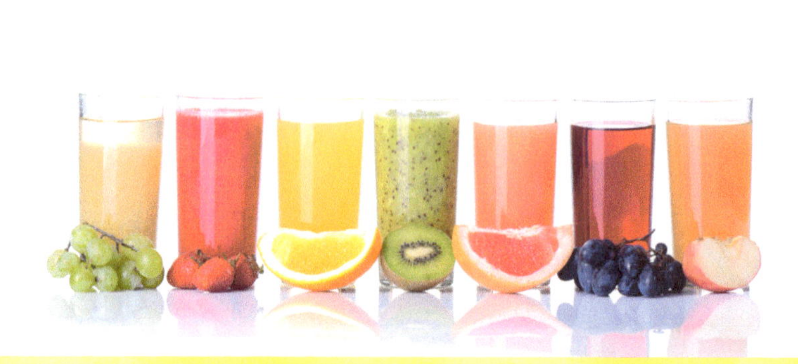

47. Pepper-carrot juice (1000 ml)

Ingredients:
- 1 red pepper
- 3 medium carrots
- 1 large apple
- 1 lemon
- 300 ml water

Preparation:
1. Wash the peppers, remove the seeds and cut into large pieces.
2. Peel the carrots and cut them into pieces.
3. Wash the apple, remove the core and cut into large pieces.
4. Halve the lemon and squeeze out the juice.
5. Put the prepared ingredients and water into a blender.
6. Mix everything until smooth.
7. Serve cold.

This recipe makes about 1000 ml of fresh pepper-carrot juice, which is rich in vitamin C and beta-carotene and supports the immune system and skin health.

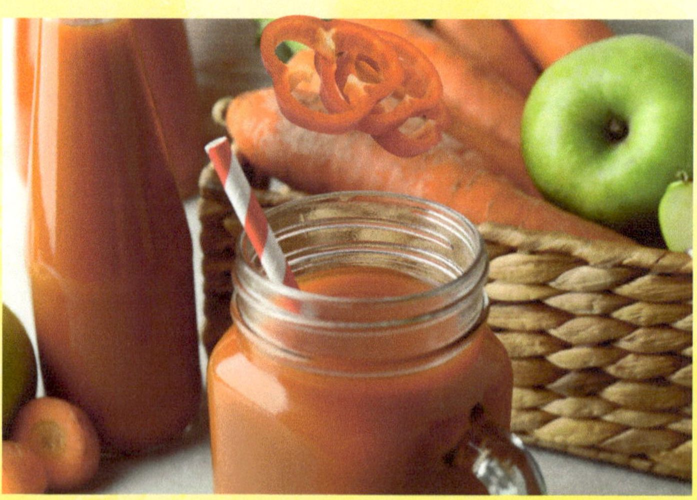

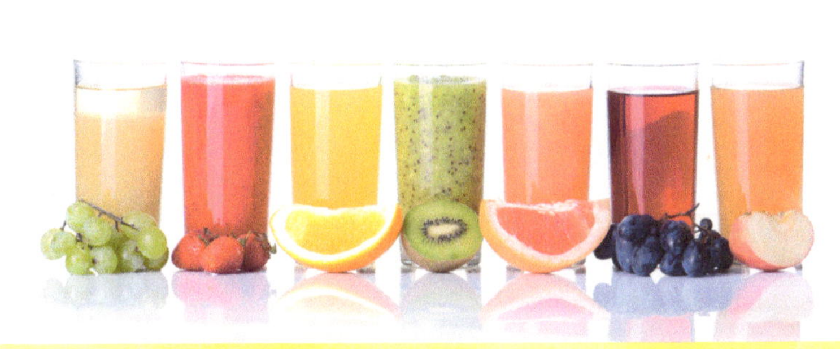

48. Apple-spinach juice (1000 ml)

Ingredients:
- 2 large apples
- 2 handfuls of fresh spinach
- 1 lemon
- 1 piece of ginger (approx. 2 cm)
- 300 ml water

Preparation:
1. Wash the apples, remove the cores and cut into large pieces.
2. Wash the fresh spinach thoroughly.
3. Halve the lemon and squeeze out the juice.
4. Peel the ginger and cut it into small pieces.
5. Put all prepared ingredients and water into a blender.
6. Mix everything until smooth.
7. Serve cold.

This recipe makes about 1000 ml of apple spinach juice, which is rich in nutrients thanks to the green leafy vegetables and fruits and strengthens the immunity.

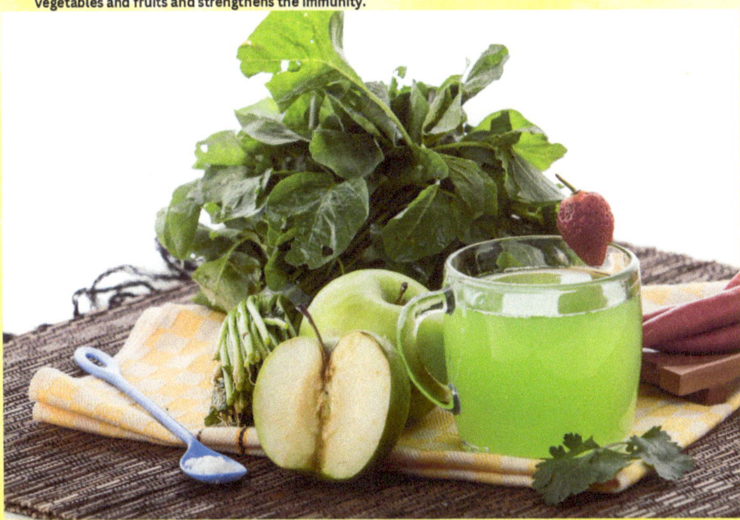

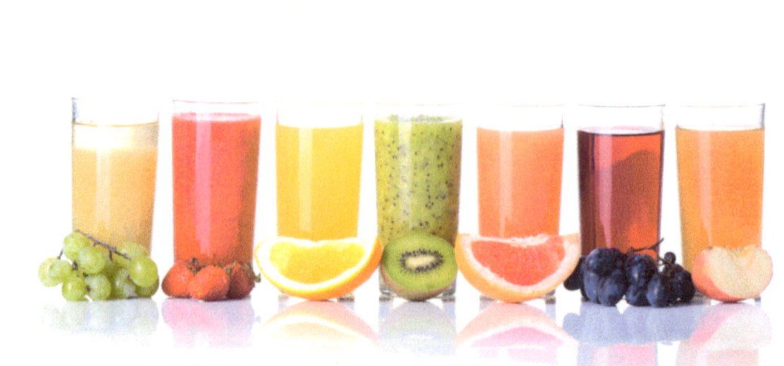

49.-50. Hydration and electrolyte juices

Keep your body optimally hydrated and balanced with our hydration and electrolyte juices. These juices are carefully formulated to support your body's fluid balance and quickly replenish lost electrolytes.

With ingredients like potassium-rich coconut water, sodium-rich cucumber, hydrating watermelon and invigorating lemon, they deliver the perfect blend of hydration and minerals.

Ideal after exercise, on hot days or simply to meet your daily fluid needs - these juices provide refreshing and healthy hydration that will make you feel good all around.

Enjoy the natural thirst quencher that invigorates your body while providing balance.

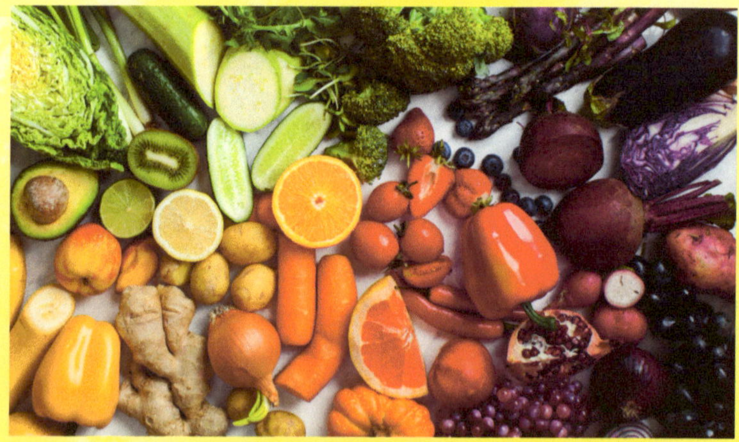

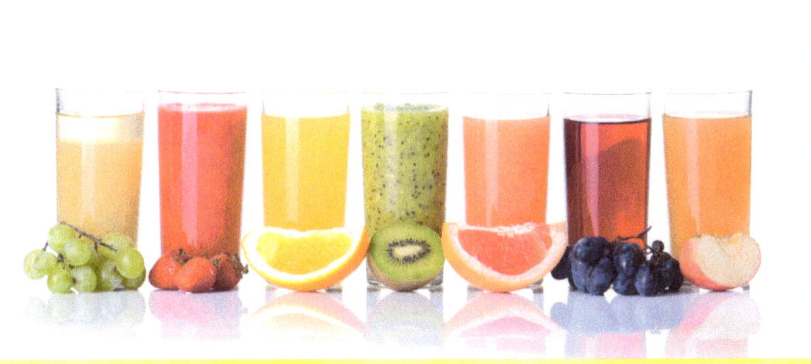

49. Watermelon Coconut Juice (1000 ml)

Ingredients:
- 500 g watermelon (without seeds)
- 300 ml coconut water
- Juice of 1 lime
- 5–6 fresh mint leaves

Preparation:
1. Cut the watermelon into large pieces.
2. Halve the lime and squeeze out the juice.
3. Wash the fresh mint leaves.
4. Place the watermelon in a blender along with the coconut water, lime juice and mint leaves.
5. Blend everything until smooth.
6. Strain the juice if a finer texture is desired.
7. Serve cold.

This recipe makes about 1000 ml of watermelon coconut juice, which is refreshing and optimally hydrates the body thanks to the natural electrolytes in the watermelon and coconut water.

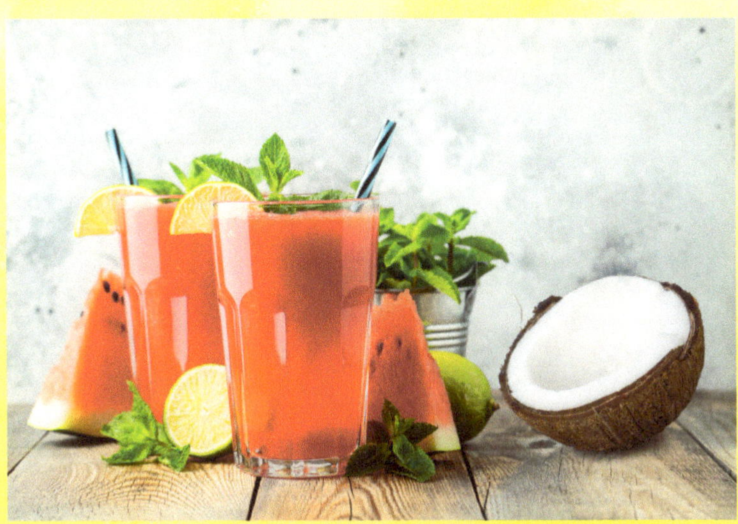

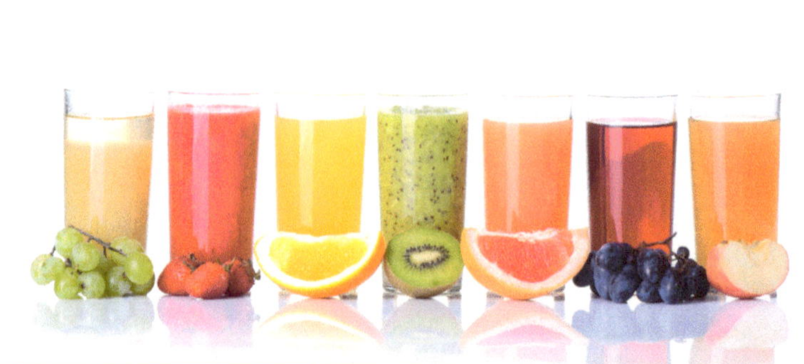

50. Cucumber-lemon juice (1000 ml)

Ingredients:
- 1 large cucumber
- 1 lemon
- 1 large apple
- 5–6 fresh mint leaves
- 200 ml water

Preparation:
1. Wash the cucumber thoroughly and cut into large pieces.
2. Halve the lemon and squeeze out the juice.
3. Wash the apple, core it and cut it into pieces.
4. Wash the fresh mint leaves.
5. Put all prepared ingredients together with the water into a blender.
6. Mix everything until smooth.
7. Serve cold.

This recipe makes about 1000 ml of cucumber and lemon juice, which is light and refreshing and ideal for supporting hydration and balancing fluid levels.

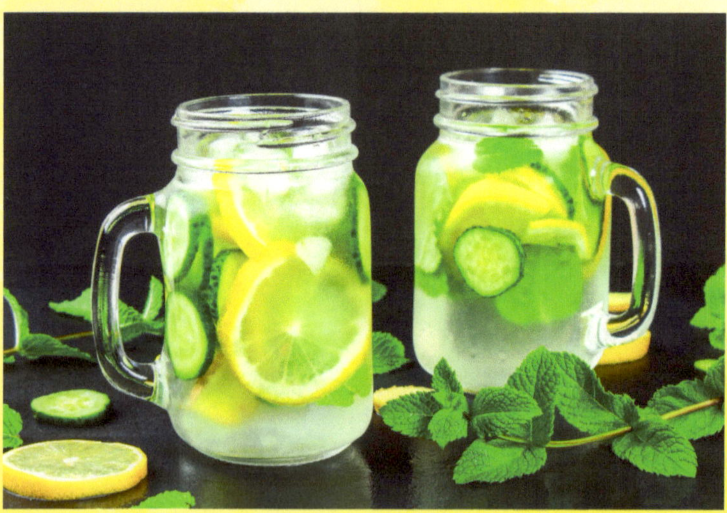

www.ingramcontent.com/pod-product-compliance
Lightning Source LLC
Chambersburg PA
CBHW040231240726
48664CB00001B/93